8/10/15
31 oct 15
u/16
22.11.21.

KT-416-172

Please return or renew this item WA(
by the last date shown. You may
return items to any East Sussex
Library. You may renew books
by telephone or the internet.

East Sussex
County Council

0345 60 80 195 for renewals
0345 60 80 196 for enquiries

Library and Information Services
eastsussex.gov.uk/libraries

04037056

Keeping Mum

CARING FOR SOMEONE
WITH DEMENTIA

MARIANNE TALBOT

HAY HOUSE

Australia • Canada • Hong Kong • India
South Africa • United Kingdom • United States

First published and distributed in the United Kingdom by:
Hay House UK Ltd, 292B Kensal Rd, London W10 5BE. Tel: (44) 20 8962 1230; Fax: (44) 20 8962 1239. www.hayhouse.co.uk

Published and distributed in the United States of America by:
Hay House, Inc., PO Box 5100, Carlsbad, CA 92018-5100. Tel: (1) 760 431 7695 or (800) 654 5126; Fax: (1) 760 431 6948 or (800) 650 5115. www.hayhouse.com

Published and distributed in Australia by:
Hay House Australia Ltd, 18/36 Ralph St, Alexandria NSW 2015. Tel: (61) 2 9669 4299; Fax: (61) 2 9669 4144. www.hayhouse.com.au

Published and distributed in the Republic of South Africa by:
Hay House SA (Pty), Ltd, PO Box 990, Witkoppen 2068. Tel./Fax: (27) 11 467 8904. www.hayhouse.co.za

Published and distributed in India by:
Hay House Publishers India, Muskaan Complex, Plot No.3, B-2, Vasant Kunj, New Delhi – 110 070. Tel: (91) 11 4176 1620; Fax: (91) 11 4176 1630. www.hayhouse.co.in

Distributed in Canada by:
Raincoast, 9050 Shaughnessy St, Vancouver, BC V6P 6E5. Tel: (1) 604 323 7100; Fax: (1) 604 323 2600

Although the author and publisher have made every effort to ensure the accuracy and completeness of information contained in this book, we assume no responsibility for errors, inaccuracies, omissions or any inconsistency herein.

A catalogue record for this book is available from the British Library.

ISBN 978-1-84850-291-8

Printed and bound in Great Britain by
CPI Group (UK) Ltd, Croydon, CR0 4YY

Contents

About the Author

Marianne Talbot cared for her parents from 1995, when a stroke rendered her father mentally incapable overnight, until 2009 when her mother died, having had Alzheimer's for 10 years. Marianne chronicled the five years her mum lived with her in the popular blog she wrote for *Saga* magazine online. The blog forms the basis of this book.

Marianne worked throughout the time she cared for her parents, as Director of Studies in Philosophy at Oxford University's Department for Continuing Education, where she is in charge of the university's 'outreach' for philosophy, including their very popular online courses.

At 15, however, Marianne was thrown out of school for truancy and disruption. She joined the 'hippie trail', travelling through Iran, Afghanistan, Pakistan and India before spending three years in Australia. She then travelled back through Africa. At 25 she started an Open University foundation course. It was during this she discovered philosophy. She was an undergraduate at the University of London, Bedford College, from 1982 to 1985, after which she moved to Corpus Christi College, Oxford to do graduate work. She taught for Pembroke College, Oxford from 1987 to 1990 and for Brasenose College, Oxford from 1990 to 2000 before taking up her current position in 2001.

From 1996 to 1999, as chair of the National Forum of Values for Education and the Community, Marianne was in charge of the spiritual, moral, social and cultural development of pupils aged 5 to 19 in English schools.

Marianne loves teaching. In 2009 a podcast of one of her lectures, 'A Romp Through the History of Philosophy', became a global number one on iTunes U (the University of iTunes). In 2010 a second podcast, 'The Nature of Argument', also became a global number one. Together they have been downloaded more than 3 million times. Marianne is tickled pink to think that people from all over the world can listen to, and watch, her lectures. You can find them here: http://www.philosophy.ox.ac.uk/podcasts.

In her spare time Marianne likes to keep fit. She cycles, swims and walks. She loves reading, especially detective novels, and the theatre, especially Shakespeare.

Foreword

by Imelda Redmond CBE
CEO Carers UK

I first met Marianne when she, at rather short notice, agreed to appear on stage at a political party Conference in 2009 for a debate on ageing and care. She describes the experience in her own words in this book, but what she doesn't say is just what an impact she had there, and continues to have, as an advocate for carers. As she does in this book, she spoke frankly and powerfully about her experiences of caring, and sent a clear message to that audience – that carers aren't a small group of do-gooders who we can pat on the head and then forget about. Having close friends or relatives who need our care and support can, and will, happen to all of us.

There are six million people in the UK who, in different ways, are living Marianne's story, as they care, unpaid, for elderly or disabled loved ones. Just as ageing is a fact of life, so is caring, and the stark reality is that, with an ageing population, *we will all care* at some point in our lives, or need care ourselves.

Yet our society and our public services have not yet caught up. At Carers UK, our research estimates that carers' contribution is the equivalent of £87 billion each year, but despite this staggering contribution, what carers do is largely unrecognized and undervalued. Our public services would not cope without carers, yet, like Marianne, too many families find that, when they need them, the services are not there to back them up – too inflexible, unreliable or simply not good enough quality. As a result, many carers are caring without the right support and are being pushed to breaking point – forced to give up their jobs, risking ill-health and sometimes poverty. It is time that our society and our politicians listen to the experiences of carers like Marianne, and give carers a better deal.

Part of the problem is that, unless you have lived through caring for a loved one, it is almost impossible to imagine what it is like. Being a carer is to be doctor, nurse, taxi (or ambulance) driver, pharmacist, physiotherapist, counsellor, cook, cleaner, accountant ... the list goes on. But on top of all these tasks and an often grinding battle with bureaucracy, you have to cope with the changes in your closest relationships, loneliness, grief, worry and the loss of your own freedom.

In this book, Marianne tells her and her mum's story, honestly – with all the frustration, despair, satisfaction and joy of being a carer. Her experiences will be a revelation to those who haven't cared for a loved one yet, and will be of huge comfort and help to carers, who will laugh and cry with it all, and know that they are not alone.

Acknowledgements

The word 'piglet', used throughout this book for the person being cared for, comes from Hugh Marriott's wonderful book *The Selfish Pig's Guide to Caring**. It stands for **P**erson **I G**ive **L**ove and **E**ndless **T**herapy to'. I think it conveys just the right combination of love and exasperation. Thank you, Hugh, for letting me use it.

Anita Ljubic, thank you for your unfailing willingness and good humour. Thank you, Andrej, for making Mum so happy, and Sinisa for lending them to me. Thank you also to Carol and Albert.

The wonderful people at the Willows day care know exactly how much I relied on them: a very big thank you. The same to everyone at the special transport service, especially Ray, everyone at Shotover, and everyone at Limes. A special thank you to Marion Collins, our care manager.

The training sessions at the Cowley Road Carers' Centre were invaluable. Through you I met the wonderful Hubert and Phoebe. Thank you. Everyone at the Headington Care Home was fantastic: thank you Elisa, and all of you for everything you did for Mum (and me). Thank you also to our GP, Gordon Gancz, and to all his brilliant receptionists. You made my life much easier.

---

*Marriott, Hugh, *The Selfish Pig's Guide to Caring* (Polperro Heritage Press, 2003)

Thank you to everyone in Cheshire who made it possible for Mum to live independently for so long. Lynne, Anita and Christine, thank you. John and Rosemary, Gordon and Elvina, Jean and John and all Mum's other Poynton friends, thank you.

Thank you to my colleagues at Oxford University's Department of Continuing Education and TALL. A special thank you to Philip Healy. Many thanks to members of the OUDCE Philosophical Society, especially committee members past and present.

Without the people at *Saga* this book wouldn't have happened. Thank you especially to Melody, Andy, Chris, Emma, Katy and all the readers of the blog (especially Bill!).

Joanna Foster, Felicity, Ian, Ollie and Rob Steadman, Philippa Morrison, Susan Quilliam, Joelle Mann and John Shirley: how often you made everything possible. Thank you for your friendship, and for opening your arms to Mum.

Finally, there's my family. In particular, Ian and Betty. Thank you. You were absolute rocks. Christopher, Judy and Richard: thanking you doesn't seem right; Mum, after all, was your mum too, she adored us all, and would, I'm sure, be proud of us for the way we managed her final years. I hope that if you read this you will recognize Mum and, if reading it prompts tears, that they are tears of happiness.

– Marianne Talbot
December 2010

Introduction

In late 2006, life was full. I was a trustee of the Girls' Day School Trust, I was Director of Studies in Philosophy at Oxford University's Department for Continuing Education, I was writing *An Introduction to Bioethics for Scientists* for Cambridge University Press, and I was Tawny Owl for a local Brownie Pack.

I was also caring for Mum.

Mum was then 86. In 1999 she had been diagnosed with Alzheimer's. She came to live with me in 2003. At first life was relatively easy. Mum could be left alone. She could also be taken out. She'd come to my lectures, to friends' dinner and lunch parties, and she loved going to the cinema, the theatre and the opera.

She was also able to help in the house (though 'help' was not always how I thought of it!). We went shopping and did the housework together, the ironing basket was empty, the silver shone and the garden had never looked better. Life was good. It was a darn sight better than it had been caring for her from a distance: what a recipe for anxiety, guilt and worry *that* had been.

By 2006, though, this happy situation was long over. I still occasionally left her alone. But I was plagued by guilt and worry. She could still come out with me. But I spent my whole time watching her. She still came to my lectures. But this was entirely thanks to my wonderful students; particularly members of the Philosophical Society.

At home, life was fraught. Social Services had become involved. Mum was going to day care. The house was never my own. It was increasingly difficult to keep the balls in the air.

It was at this point I added to my 'to do' list a monthly blog for *Saga* magazine online. Was I mad?

No. The blog added to my ridiculous workload, but writing it was incredibly therapeutic.

If I was stressed, anxious or angry, I expressed it in the blog. If I was sad, depressed or worried, writing the blog was comforting. If something funny happened, or my love for Mum felt particularly strong, into the blog it would go. If I had had a run-in with a jobsworth, where better to vent my fury than to the blog?

To my huge pleasure the readers – mostly other carers – lapped it up. Very soon the web-editor, Melody, asked me if I would do a weekly rather than a monthly blog. I was happy to do so. I derived huge comfort from the messages left by other carers, especially those saying they found the blog helpful.

It was like having a group of supportive friends in whom to confide. Friends, furthermore, who I knew would understand. It is only if you have cared for someone with dementia that you can really understand what it is like. Others sympathize, understand intellectually, commiserate and tell you you're doing a great job. But they do not understand the visceral fear, anxiety, loneliness and fury that are part and parcel of being responsible for someone whose mind is fragmenting.

Nor do they understand the logistical nightmare of dealing day in, day out with someone whose memory span is literally 3 seconds long.

People often think that caring for someone with dementia must be like caring for a child. This comparison is misleading. Extremely misleading.

A child who is able to walk is cognitively streets ahead of someone whose dementia has reached the final stage. A friend of mine once – very kindly – visited Mum with his two small dogs. Mum, adoring animals, was delighted.

My marvellous friend, despite knowing Mum had end-stage Alzheimer's, couldn't wrap his mind around the fact that, as the dogs disappeared behind the sofa, they ceased to exist for her. He described to me in wonder how, every time they reappeared, her delight was as if she had no idea they were there. This, of course, was exactly the situation: she didn't have any idea they *were* there when she could no longer *see* them there.

The human memory is extraordinary. If it works it goes unnoticed. The temporary loss of a particular word or name is momentarily frustrating, and as we get older memory lapses become more frequent. But normal age-related memory loss is as nothing compared to the profound loss that comes with dementia.

Imagine not being able to hold a conversation (you can't remember the last thing said). Imagine not being able to learn anything new (including the location of the loo in your own home). Imagine not being able to remember the names of your children, or how many children you have. Imagine not knowing where you are, why you are there or who anyone else is. Imagine not knowing who *you* are.

Imagine all this and thank God for your memory.

Our identities, our very sense of who we are, are spun from a web of memories: memories we share with siblings, partners, children and friends, memories of what we have felt and believed at different times of our lives, memories of things we are proud of and things that make us blush with shame. If we lose our memories there is a deep and profound sense in which we lose ourselves.

If you are caring, or have cared, for someone with dementia, this will be familiar to you. You will know the desperate sadness of watching someone you love descend into this pit, a pit in which they are isolated from any, and every, other human being. Even from you.

But you will also know that the stripping away of a person's memory is *not* the disintegration of the whole person. Something is left.

Until the day of her death, Mum was still *Mum*. She had no idea who I was, but her eyes lit up when she saw me. She couldn't produce a meaningful sentence, but she still understood – and loved – a bear hug. She would eat the daffodils I gave her for Mother's Day, but her enjoyment of food was intact.

I am proud of having brought Mum to live with me for her final years. Caring for her leaves me a legacy of love that will last until the final years of *my* life. When she died I felt I had done everything I could to make the end of her life as comfortable, and meaningful, as possible.

If you are a carer, this is what you are doing. It is, I believe, one of the most important ways someone can spend their time. You are doing everything you can to make the most of the life of another human being.

Amazingly, when you put 'carer' on your CV it won't impress anyone. In our society people are more impressed by your pay packet than your willingness to care for someone you love. But you know and I know that this, really, is where it is at. Be proud.

Now the blog has become – with the help of the wonderful people at Hay House – this book. In it you will find some new blogs and, at the end of each blog, a short tip or commentary. I have included my popular short piece for *Saga* magazine 'Marianne's Tips for Carers'. There are also short chapters on the practicalities of, firstly, money, property and the law, and secondly Social Services, health and welfare. With some trepidation, I have included a short chapter on 'Carers' Fury': you will know what I mean. There are also lists of addresses you might find useful.

I should be very happy if the practical suggestions in this book make life easier for you. I should cringe, though, if you thought that in offering such tips I am setting myself up as an expert carer. All I can justifiably claim to be, after 14 years, is an *experienced* carer. One with friends who are also experienced carers and who have been happy to share with me tips that they have found useful. I pass these tips on to you hoping they will help.

Both my beloved parents, having lived long, productive and enjoyable lives, are now dead. My caring duties are over. Many of you are not in this position. Some of you – caring for partners or children – may never be in this position. I feel for you from the bottom of my heart.

But I know that you won't begrudge me my freedom. I promise you I'll use it well. I also promise I shan't forget you. I shall do everything in my power to promote the cause of carers: if I can help *you,* or an organization you belong to, be in touch at the address below or on the Keeping Mum website www.keepingmum.org.uk

Marianne Talbot
c/o Hay House
marianne.talbot@conted.ox.ac.uk

THE BLOG

In the Beginning

When Mum set fire to the microwave (baking a potato on 'high' for an hour) I knew the time had come. On this occasion the neighbours were there, but what if they hadn't been? She had been diagnosed with Alzheimer's four years before, but was still – just – managing independently. Obviously this was becoming untenable.

So three years ago my mum moved in with me.

That makes it sound easy. It was actually a nightmare of buying and selling houses, spitting rows with brothers and sisters and unwelcome discoveries about the fact Mum hadn't really been managing at all. But this was after the making of The Decision.

I didn't take lightly the idea of her living with me. I read every book on Alzheimer's I could lay my hands on. I spoke at length to Mum's consultant. I trawled the carers' websites and I played devil's advocate with myself. I knew that if I resented her it wouldn't work.

I reflected seriously on my 'non-negotiables' (things like solitude, swimming, working and walking), wanting to know how

1

I would get them consistently with Mum living with me. I bore in mind the fact that a time would come when I couldn't leave Mum alone. How would I get my non-negotiables then? I also thought about Mum's non-negotiables (independence, dignity, a social life and fun) and whether I could provide them.

I considered, of course, how we would manage with the things that would – from long experience – rub the other up the wrong way. We'd always got on extremely well, but there had always been spits and spats.

When I invited her to live with me it was because I really believed I could do it. I remember thinking, in fact, that it wasn't so much a matter of believing I could do it, as making the commitment that I *would* do it. Then the similarity with the marriage vows struck me – 'til death us do part' and all that. Oh dear.

I won't pretend there haven't been tears, both for Mum and me, but overall it has worked brilliantly. She's a lovely old bat, my mum. She's endlessly cheerful, she loves everyone and everything, and she's so open to novelty she puts some younger people to shame.

I sometimes remember with a shock that this story won't have a happy ending. When that happens I'll mourn her twice – once as the delightful, charming and completely dotty old dear she is now, and once, when the shock has worn off, for the doughty, practical, intelligent woman she once was.

But I won't dwell on that – got to get her up for day care.

Caring from a distance and worried about your piglet leaving gas appliances on? Get an isolation valve fitted. It isn't terribly expensive (£40 when I did it) and gives huge peace of mind. Meals on wheels and central heating are essential, though, or your piglet's life won't be worth living.

In case you missed the Acknowledgements 'piglet' is short for **Person I Give** Love and Endless Therapy to'. See *The Selfish Pig's Guide to Caring** by Hugh Marriott. Completely brilliant!

Mum-Time

Off to the ophthalmologist yesterday. I knew it would be a waste of time. I'm glad our optician cares enough to get Mum seen to, but I wish it didn't involve hospital visits. Mum's short-term memory span is 3 seconds. On the 10-minute walk to the bus we have the same conversation 20 times: 'Where are we going?', 'To the ophthalmologist.' 'Why?' 'To have your eyes checked', 'But there's nothing wrong with my eyes.' 'That's what we are hoping to confirm.'

On the bus it's another 20 times (to the bemusement of the woman behind), then again on the walk to the hospital, and again in the waiting room. Then we do it all again in reverse.

This can be relaxing: once I've said whatever I'm going to say, I just keep saying it. Totally undemanding. The very predictability of it allows me to continue my own train of thought, whilst Mum feels that I am companionably responding to her. When this is happening such trips can be fun – warm, close and life-enhancing.

But if I am stressed, the exercise is rather different. Invariably I try to rush her. But Mum does not do fast. If I speak quickly, she doesn't hear. If I move quickly she gets confused. If I get exasperated, she feels bewildered and starts to look lost. This is anything but fun. I feel guilty, Mum feels useless and it can take the evening to recover.

I am becoming good at slowing myself down for Mum, especially when rushing would be counterproductive (i.e. nearly always). It must look rather comical – I dash around like a maniac

*Marriott, Hugh, *The Selfish Pig's Guide to Caring* (Polperro Heritage Press, 2003)

until Mum is in sight then I suddenly s l o w d o w n until, out of her sight again, I speed up. Like one of those cartoon characters.

I have discovered a fund of patience that I didn't know I had since Mum came. When I succeed in slowing down, then however stressed I am I actually start to *feel* less stressed. I set off with Mum to go somewhere, for example, feeling desperate at having to spend the time doing it, but then I find myself entering into her world.

This is a world in which every flower is to be gloried at, every neat hedge to be approved of, every silver car to be admired. Every passer-by is greeted and smiled at, every child chucked under the chin and every cat stroked.

I enjoy this world so much that it is quite frightening to think that if Mum hadn't come to live with me I might never have discovered it.

Before Mum moved in with me, the telephone was her lifeline. Often, though, she'd fail to put it back on the hook. This racked up bills for calls of several hours' duration. I found BT extraordinarily helpful: whenever I explained the situation they agreed to refund her. Worth a try!

Social Services to the Rescue

In London for the day with a carer booked until 6 p.m. By 5 p.m. I had spent an hour and a half in the same traffic jam and saw no likelihood of early release. I rang the carer (thank goodness for mobiles). But she had to get home. One neighbour was out but the other – who has two children – plugged the gap (an hour and a half's worth). Came home to find Mum in her element, in a tangle of arms and legs, tickling toddlers.

These relatively small crises are nothing compared to those I had before Mum moved in. Compared to caring from a distance, having Mum living with me is a doddle. I used to feel permanently guilty, not least because Mum was lonely, but mostly because I worried about her. This worry was usually unfounded, but occasionally it reached fever pitch.

Once, for example, I was away at a conference. Checking my answer-phone late in the evening I found an impassioned plea from Mum's vicar, telling me her alarm was ringing and she wasn't answering it, or the telephone. He had been to the house but all the curtains were closed. It was then midnight. I rang the vicar (poor man), but no answer. Heart thumping I considered whether to ring the police, the Social Services and/or her doctor. I went for the Social Services and was amazed that they answered the phone on the second ring, agreed to send someone out immediately, and said they'd phone me back as soon as they had news.

Heart fluttering, I settled down to wait.

Twenty minutes later (!) they rang back. When they had got to the house the police were there, with two neighbours and the vicar. This lot trooped upstairs and went into Mum's room, the alarm still ringing. Waking up, she turned on them a beatific smile and said how pleased she was to see them. She simply hadn't heard the alarm.

A happy ending. But it was incidents like that that made me realize that Mum really couldn't go on living alone, 200 miles away from me (and neither of us with a car). Since she has lived with me the guilt and the worry have largely gone, to be replaced by organizational angst and occasional frustration.

But thank goodness for the Social Services. Both where Mum lived before and here, they really are marvellous. They are usually efficient, always kind, sometimes saint-like and extremely knowledgeable. It is easy to carp – especially at the end of one's tether (and carers spend a lot of time there) – but without them the job would simply be undoable.

One of the joys of caring, actually, is meeting so many people who devote their lives to helping others, cheerfully and competently. Humbling, really.

If your piglet is like Mum, they are too trusting. If you are caring from a distance be aware that anyone coming to the door will be invited in. If they are selling something – gas, windows – your piglet will certainly buy. Keep a beady eye on bank statements (for which you'll need an LPA: see pages 236–37)

The Delights of Day Care

When the idea of day care was first mooted, I was sceptical. I didn't think Mum would go for it at all. My image of day care was of elderly people in silent rows, television blaring, waiting to be collected by their carer (or the grim reaper: would it matter?).

But the situation was becoming unmanageable. Mum sat alone day after day whilst I worked in the next room. When she was able to amuse herself this was fine, but her ability to do that was clearly on its way out. She had lost faith in her needlework, spending more time unpicking it than working on it (and having to thread a needle for her every 5 minutes was driving me up the wall). Initially, too, she didn't mind reading the same parts of the same book over and over, but her grasp of even the most tenuous thread of a story had disappeared. She had been reduced to sitting doing nothing – or, as she touchingly said when asked: 'I am thinking.'

So day care started to seem attractive, not least in alleviating my guilt at not being more attentive.

On her first day I nervously went with her. But having served the coffee, they proceeded to do a crossword (on a large whiteboard). What fun! I didn't know whether to be proud or embarrassed. Mum yelled every answer – more or less correctly – the minute the clue was read out. No one else got a look-in. She was beaming: she always was good with words. An hour later, unnoticed, I slunk out.

So it has continued. She has completely blossomed. The vacant look that was beginning to stalk her features has gone. She is animated, interested and interesting. Her social skills – not a jot affected by the Alzheimer's – are again in full use. She flirts with the men, makes confidantes of the women, is endlessly charming to the professional carers, and generally enhances any gathering she's in. She likes everyone and everyone seems to like her.

Her days are now varied. Some days she has to get up early to be fetched by the special bus, and other days she can lie in as long as she likes (my mum can sleep for England). On the days she's at home she'll happily read the paper (the same paragraph again and again), do the ironing (I haven't ironed so much as a handkerchief since she moved in), and chat to the cat.

I credit the people who run the day care, and the wonderful communities they create (from some of the most unpromising material imaginable), with keeping my mum alive in the most important sense – her spirit.

If your piglet goes to day care, use an exercise book as a 'log' book. Note when they are collected, and dropped off, and ask the staff to jot down what they had for lunch, what their mood was like, and things like coughs, bad temper, loose bowels or exceptional lucidity.

Caring from a Distance

Not having to care from a distance is wonderful. I used to be constantly worrying, panicking or feeling guilty. Now I know where Mum is, what she's doing and whether she's eating, sleeping, warm or cheerful. It's fantastic!

I'd known for ages Mum shouldn't be living alone. She was a danger to herself and, given that she lived in a terrace of cottages, to others. She was also desperately lonely.

Mum boasts she can make friends anywhere. She's right. Nearly everyone takes to her. She is interested in everyone and everything and can make even the most boring person feel fascinating.

But during the last couple of years of living alone she felt vulnerable. I am not sure why. She didn't seem to be aware of her confusion or loss of memory. But that might have been a ploy – she definitely had (and has) strategies for hiding it, so she must be aware at some level. Maybe it was just that she was getting older? Anyway, where once, if loneliness threatened, she would have taken herself to the cinema or to see friends or family, by then she was just staying at home feeling lonely.

Knowing this, I was ringing her whenever possible for a chat. But this meant that I felt guilty whenever I didn't have time to chat. Sometimes, too, the phone would ring and ring. Then I'd start to worry about where she was and what she was doing. I'd imagine her wandering lost having tried to get to the village. Or I'd imagine her lying ill in bed unable to call for help. I would then ring and ring and ring, panic rising, until finally she answered, having been in the garden or somewhere equally unthreatening.

Then there were the logistics of trying to arrange, from a distance, the life of an increasingly demented old lady.

Getting Mum to the dentist, for example, was a triumph of my organizational skills, the dentist's good nature and Mum's willingness. Mum wouldn't, of course, remember the appointment (or to look at her diary), so I had to keep a diary for her.

At the appropriate moment I would ring, tell her to put her coat on, then tell her to go to the village. At least habit usually took her

8

in the right direction. Then I'd ring the dentist's receptionist, who would look out for her. Sometimes Mum would just disappear, to turn up a couple of hours later, having been goodness knows where. Then the whole process would have to be repeated when I'd rearranged the appointment.

You might think that bringing her to live with me was a major decision: in my experience caring from a distance is *not* the easy option.

> Mum insisted she could clean the house herself. But even if she could, she wasn't doing it. I persuaded her to accept a cleaner from Age Concern (now Age UK) on the grounds that her advanced age qualified her for help. Christine became a friend to Mum, and a source of reliable comfort to me. Try your local Age UK to see if they offer such a service.

Postal Scams

When Mum lived independently, a major difficulty was dealing with her increasing inability to think things through. She was always a trusting person (because she was herself so trustworthy, I think), but she became even more trusting.

At one point whenever I phoned her, she would tell me she'd had a letter (often from Canada) saying she had won a prize, or the lottery, or had been sent a present from abroad. She would excitedly tell me about the promised riches – £10,000, £20,000 or something 'to the value of' such amounts. She was completely taken in.

I started by tentatively saying she should ignore the letters, that it was probably a scam. That backfired because, understanding that I disapproved, she started herself saying they were probably a scam. But I could hear the excitement still in her voice. It was obvious that she intended to do whatever they wanted. She just wasn't going to tell me about it.

So I suggested that she send me the letters and I would make sure she got the prize if she had won one. She did send a couple, and sure enough they were a scam: 'Send us £20 to cover costs and we will send a cheque by return.' So *this* is what all those odd £20 and £10 cheques were covering (I already operated her bank account by this time). She was spending a *fortune*.

It also explained all the tat Mum had been collecting. Those cheap trinkets in her bedside drawer were the 'pure gold cufflinks' and 'precious diamond and pearl earrings' she was paying for out of her hard-earned pension.

So I arranged to have all her mail forwarded to me. Within a month I had no fewer than 60 of these letters. Sixty! Among them were offers of forecasts of her future, charms that would protect her from harm, numerous lottery wins and as many 'prizes'. All asked her to send cheques for amounts varying from £10 to £100.

According to Mum's postman, all elderly people living alone get these letters regularly. He hated delivering them, and frequently warned 'his' elderly people not to respond to them, but he didn't think anyone listened.

Sometimes my faith in human nature takes a real knock. How can people *do* this? If you care for someone from a distance, do keep an eye on their mail – you may find the same thing is happening to them.

If you're caring from a distance and you suspect your piglet is getting these scam letters, arrange for the post office to send their mail to you. Then send the letters to the Trading Standards people. No idea what they do with them, but you'll feel better.

Postal Shenanigans

As Mum was wasting so much money on postal scams I completed a form at the post office (you can also do this online) and paid a fee to have her post redirected to me. It was easy.

Well, I say it was easy. If you're redirecting the mail of someone with dementia it can get more complicated.

When I was working at home one day, the phone rang. It was Paul, Mum's postman. He was worried. He had been joking with Mum about the redirection of her post and she had claimed to know nothing about it.

Well, I had certainly told her. Asked her, indeed. I wouldn't redirect her post without her permission. But the fact Mum had agreed to it a few weeks back was, of course, irrelevant. She remembered nothing of our conversation, or the reason for her post being redirected to me.

I reassured Paul and took the opportunity to warn him that she'd soon be moving, and that she'd probably deny knowledge of that, too. But whilst Paul was on, I mentioned to him that I had been wondering how to get Mum's 'real' mail back to her.

My original intention had been to post it. I expect you'll see the catch.

But I didn't want Mum to feel suddenly bereft of post. She had, after all, been getting so much. I wonder to what extent these scam letters succeed because getting post is such a pleasure to elderly people who live alone?

Paul immediately said that he and his mate in the sorting office could deal with that. If I just packed Mum's 'real' mail into an envelope and addressed it to her c/o him at the sorting office, he'd make sure Mum got it during his normal round.

Paul also tells me he keeps an eye on Mum, together with all 'his' other old people. He gets to know their routines, and if something is out of the ordinary he hangs around until he is sure they're OK.

What a star! Quite the opposite of a jobsworth don't you think? Warms the cockles of one's heart.

Actually all the people in Mum's village are fantastic. The shopkeepers, for example, let her take goods without paying (she always claims to have no money), trusting me to pay when I come in. They'll also ring me if she comes in having forgotten where she was going.

This can be very useful. If she has an appointment, the best I can do by telephone is get her out of the door with her coat on. After that she's on her own.

Thank goodness she's surrounded by kindness.

> If your piglet doesn't live with you, introduce yourself to their neighbours and the local shopkeepers. You may discover some distressing things (such as the amount of help they're giving your piglet). But it's better to know, and it's useful to be aware of people who have already demonstrated their willingness to help.

Fellow-Travellers

Like most carers, I have learned everything I know by trial and error (mainly error). So when the local Carers' Centre (wonderful organization) asked if I'd like to go on a workshop on Caring for People with Dementia, I jumped at it, even before they told me they'd pay for Mum's care while I attended.

But what an eye-opener. Heart-rending. One chap, caring for his wife, was ridden with guilt because every time he left the house she clung to him and cried. A woman whose husband had recently gone into a home because she could no longer cope was also guilt-ridden because she felt she was deserting him. Another woman, whose husband was aggressive and occasionally violent, was clearly hanging on by her fingernails. One woman, obviously herself suffering the onset of dementia, was still caring for her severely demented husband.

I felt guilty, too, when I had to confess that my mum is not only as happy as Larry, but also – relatively – fit and easy to care for. Only one other person attending was in a similar position, a man caring for his wife, who sounds just like my mum.

A couple of people, like me, were caring for parents, but most were caring for partners. One hears so much about troubled marriages that seeing 'in sickness and in health' being lived out so thoroughly is hugely touching. An elderly man doesn't expect, after a lifetime of seeing his wife cope with everything, to find himself helping her on with her support stockings, and hanging around outside the Ladies room for a woman who looks nice enough to help her go to the loo. If you want to see love in action, go to a carers' workshop.

But be warned: the more negative human emotions are also palpable. There are plenty of tears, a pall of anxiety, and manifest exhaustion. But the odd thing is that it very quickly becomes funny. The difficulties of getting an old lady out of the bath become a story that everyone enjoys (not least because they've all done it); the pig-headed stubbornness of the husband who doesn't accept he needs care becomes a fond tale that has tears of laughter running down everyone's faces; the mother who gardens by pulling up everything in sight prompts huge mirth.

It is cheering to share stories with people in the same position. Non-carers may laugh at our stories (it's the way we tell them) but their overwhelming feeling seems to be pity, which can be very isolating. I greatly enjoyed meeting other carers and will certainly go again.

Sometimes piglets are made overnight. Sometimes it takes years. Either way the focus will be on the piglet. Your transition from ordinary person to carer is likely to go unnoticed. Consciously recognizing your new status allows you properly to address your new needs and get some help. See the Resources chapter on pages 275–84.

Double Panic

Mum doesn't often get distressed. But she cannot bear children or animals, or *anyone*, actually, being hurt. Children, though, are her real concern. Despite having had four of her own without any sign of sentimentality, she no longer understands that children just *do* get upset, accidents happen, or that people just *do* hurt children. Her look of bewilderment is painful to me.

On a daily basis, therefore, I go through the newspaper removing anything that'll upset her. Have you *any idea* how many children get hurt? (A charity that should know better is using a picture of the eyes of a terrified elderly lady. This one goes straight into the bin.)

My nine-month-old godson Will spent the evening with us recently. His first time away from his mum and dad. At first he was his usual smiling self, basking in my mum's cooing. But then his mum left.

It took a minute. Then sheer panic crossed his little face and he let out a wail that must have been heard 10 miles away. Immediately Mum's face expressed a similar panic, though her wail was more restrained. I suddenly had a screaming baby and a panicking elderly woman on my hands.

Calming Mum while the baby screamed was clearly not a runner. It seemed easier to leave Mum panicking, take the baby upstairs and deal with him first.

I tried distracting him but he wouldn't even look at my offerings. I tried singing to him but felt idiotic competing with his 100-decibel wails. Eventually, deciding he was perfectly rational to cry under the circumstances, I just let him do so, stroking his back for an hour until he'd exhausted himself and gone to sleep.

Now to Mum. Well, you'd think she'd have forgotten all about it – she forgets everything else, for goodness' sake! But no she was only too agitatedly aware that there was a distressed baby in the house. The next hour was spent stroking *her* back and calming *her*.

Eventually I got her into bed and asleep, whereupon young Will, having restored himself, awoke and renewed his wailing.

Obviously, though, his energy was waning, and 30 minutes later all was calm. He obliged me by listening to my commentary on the nonsense on television, honouring me now and then with a totally disarming smile. By the time his mum returned I was in love with him again and didn't even feel insulted when, with crows of delight, he hurled himself into her arms without a backwards glance.

Your piglet will probably read the newspaper far longer than they will read books – no need to keep a story in mind. When Mum got to this point I ransacked the charity shops for picture books. This worked for quite a while. They were very cheap, too.

Fatcat and Oedipus

My cat Oedipus does not have a nice nature. Far too handy with his claws. But he's been with me since he was eight weeks old and I adore him. For 10 years I was the only human with whom he had sustained contact, and he was undoubtedly King of the Castle.

But that was in my previous house, and Mum couldn't possibly have lived there: a deathtrap of steep stairs, damp and rodents. So we moved, Oedipus and I, to a 'proper' house, to await Mum's arrival.

Trauma! The cat who happily got into his basket for the vet refused point-blank and had to be forced in. There he yowled, growled, spat and hissed as we were driven around for the hour I was advised it would take him to get thoroughly disorientated. Decanted into my new bedroom he fled under the duvet and stayed there for two weeks. His eyes, when I peered in, were huge and petrified. I felt like Cruella de Ville.

After two weeks he started to venture into the room. Then he came downstairs. Then he showed an interest in the garden. Within a month he was his old self. I even found him in a cartoon clinch with a neighbouring cat, locked in a screeching ball of claws, fur flying as they rolled into the road together.

But then Mum moved in. With Fatcat. Fatcat is well-named. She is the largest cat I have ever seen. They tell you that cats will only eat what they need. If so, Fatcat has a bit missing. She'll eat anything. Have you ever seen a cat eat fruitcake? Fatcat does. And melon. It might not be her fault: Mum's deteriorating memory meant that she only ever fed poor old Fatcat when she was herself eating. If she had a chocolate bar, so did Fatcat; if she had broccoli, so did Fatcat.

The first time Oedipus and Fatcat met was electrifying. Both puffed up hugely and issued warning rumbles. Then they circled each other in a stiff-legged walk, then each hurled itself at the other and I had to separate them with a broom. For a month or two this happened every time they met. It shocked Mum speechless every time they did it.

Then they started to ignore each other, spitting and spatting only when meeting unexpectedly. Now they can even be in the same room together, though I fear they'll never be bosom buddies.

But at least there's something like a ceasefire, and nowadays at bedtime Fatcat curls up on Mum's bed, Oedipus on mine and it can even seem quite peaceful.

You don't have to keep pets in order for your piglet to enjoy animals. Find neighbours with a dog and persuade them to let you and your piglet walk it. Trawl the neighbourhood for friendly cats, and take your walks by their house. Mum used to love the ducks on a neighbour's pond.

Bathtime

Oh dearie me, what a fright. I couldn't get Mum out of the bath last night. She's quite large (used to be 5'10", still 11 stone) and has little strength in her arms. The blasted mat didn't help. It's supposed to be non-slip, but it gives Mum just enough confidence to trust it before it slips, taking her with it.

It took us an hour and a half. That's an hour and a half in a damp, rapidly cooling bathroom for an old lady who, despite attempts to remain cheerful, is frightened and near tears. I was frightened, too, and wondering whether to call the police or the fire brigade (it now occurs to me the obvious would have been an ambulance).

First we tried our usual method (grasp front rail with left hand, side rail with right, tuck feet underneath and *heave*). The mat did for this one. Then we tried sideways, legs both over the side, pushing off with her back. Hopeless. Then we had a rest. Or she did. I was too busy warming towels to comfort her. Then we tried again.

The first time it went wrong we laughed. The second time we laughed harder. By the third time the laugh had become a manic gurgle, and after that we concentrated on stopping ourselves from crying. Mum is such a trooper. She was worried about my worry, and trying to convince me she was fine – nearly as hard as I was trying to convince her she was.

This has happened before. Recently, at the suggestion of the Social Services, we went to a mobility place to try bath aids. But Mum can't bear people to think she's anything other than fit and independent. Alerted by the questions she was asked (all of which she answered incorrectly) and the request that she sit in an empty bath with all her clothes on, she knew she was being tested, and rose to the challenge.

Asked whether she could stand up from a small stool placed in the bath, up she leapt like a Spring lamb, chortling '*Of course I can!*' Our advisor, being committed – reasonably enough – to releasing only the minimum a person can manage with, thereby assigned us the stool despite my protests that Mum would never actually use it. It now gathers dust under my bed, and bathing is becoming a major trial.

So what do I do? No point in returning to the mobility place: Mum'll do her Spring lamb act again. Give up on baths? How awful never again to enjoy a long hot bath. A larger bathroom would be nice. Dream on.

If anyone has any suggestions I should be delighted to hear …

> If you need bath appliances (or other aids) and for some reason Social Services can't help, check out the carers' chat rooms, the noticeboard at your local hospital or Carers' Centre or the notices in carers' newsletters. You'd be amazed how cheaply they're sold off by carers who no longer need them.

A Piglet Swap

We went out to dinner last Friday, Mum and I. An experiment. My friend's husband has Lewy Body Dementia [similar in some ways to the dementia of Alzheimer's and the movement problems of Parkinson's], and she and I have regular lunches to remind ourselves of when we had real lives. Last time, after the fourth glass of wine, we had a brilliant idea: Why not bring our piglets together? If they could amuse each other, we could relax.

It worked!

Mum was delighted to be out with me and her enthusiasm ran away with her. Within the first 10 minutes she commented about 100 times on their glorious view and splendid fireplace. Normally I would curl up inside. But, each time, Philippa responded – and with equal warmth! She also took in her stride Mum's offers to help (people are usually petrified for their precious china/glass/toes/children). Philippa cheerfully gave her something to do.

In the meantime I talked to my friend's husband about his work, his sons and his feelings about his situation. His memory is better than Mum's – so far – and he has more insight into his condition. My heart went out to him – Lewy Body Dementia is more disabling physically then Alzheimer's, and Martin is only 68. Life really isn't fair. But here he was holding a dinner party with his wife and apparently enjoying the role of host.

Dinner was a dream. By normal standards the conversation was Alice-in-Wonderlandish, the strawberries largely unhulled (one of Mum's jobs) and the napkins extremely well used. But it was *fun*.

For *all* of us. Philippa's buttons weren't pushed by Mum, my buttons weren't pushed by Martin. Mum and Martin expanded under the attention. Philippa and I basked in the unusual glow of having done everything right.

I suspect that real conversation often ceases when people live together. But when one of them has dementia conversation is actually impossible. Conversations depend on enough memory to be able to hold a thread. Mum's memory simply isn't up to the job, and though Martin's memory is still OK, he is difficult to understand.

When Mum and I are alone I make inane comments on whatever I'm reading so she feels we're interacting. But it can feel so patronizing. It also feels patronizing when I repeat my responses to her repeated questions. But how else is one to converse with someone who reads aloud the same sentence from the paper 20 times in 20 minutes, each time with the same air of astonishment? I sometimes think I should put in more effort, but when it actually comes to it I never do.

But it was a pleasure to concentrate on Martin for an evening. And Philippa says she enjoyed Mum. Perhaps we have finally found the secret – swap piglets!

You'd be amazed how many other people there are in your situation. If you can find some you can then brainstorm with them on how you might help each other. Does one hate cooking? One hate shopping? Swapping or pooling chores could make all the difference.

Routines

Routines are crucial to caring, in my opinion. They certainly help Mum, and they help me by making at least some things predictable. The 'getting up' routine is the one I enjoy most.

I go in about 8.40 a.m., draw the curtains and sing 'Wakey, wakey, rise and shine!' (this was my dad's morning greeting. Other women turn into their mums; I have turned into my dad). Mum mutters something like 'Um-um' and pulls the duvet closer. I lean over, kiss her and say: 'Ten minutes, then I'm going to tip you out.' 'Um-um' she says again, screwing her eyes more tightly shut.

Ten minutes later, I warn her I am about to tip her out. 'Go away,' she says. I yank the duvet off her feet and start to pull off her bedsocks. She resists, but I have her feet and can tickle them. Once her socks are off, I pull off the duvet. At this outrage she splutters 'You are a pest!' or 'What a nasty girl you are!' or 'You're a bully, you are.' I tell her that I learned my bullying skills from her, and make her sit up.

Next she has a shower. Boy, does she hate showers! But I can't bear the thought of people avoiding her because of an 'old lady' smell, so I insist. Again she tells me I am a bully, again I say I learned how to be a bully from her. (It's true. I still have mental scars from her plaiting of my hair before school.)

Then she gets dressed. Up to a point, she can dress herself. But it takes a long time, makes her tired, and results in rather exotic outfits (the best was the bra over the dress – but didn't the Princess of Wales do this once?). Every minute is punctuated by conversations identical to the ones we have every morning: 'I haven't got a handkerchief.' 'Yes, you have, it's in your sleeve.' 'Time to do your teeth.' 'Do I have to?' 'It's non-negotiable.' 'What do I do now?' 'Go downstairs and eat your cereal.'

But it is the predictability of it that ensures its smooth running. Even though she lacks a cognitive memory, Mum has, I'm sure, an emotional one, and it's routines like this that make her feel safe. We have a lot of fun as we run through our routines – she plays her allotted role and feels in charge. I know she feels good, so I feel good, too.

Ho yes! It is a fine art. I feel quite proud of myself as I usher a clean, breakfasted and cheerful Mum out to the day care bus.

People with dementia, like young children, are comforted by repetition. When trying to entertain Mum I sometimes used to bang out a simple rhythm on something (a chair arm, magazine, whatever) again and again until she joined in. She invariably did. With a huge grin. You might even buy an old toy drum, or fill some plastic containers or jars with beans to make maracas.

Story-telling

Mum used to be a great story-teller. She'd tell the same story over and over again, but everyone forgave her because it'd be newly embellished each time, and she'd tell it with such verve.

One of her favourites was about the birth of her twin brothers, Ian and Bryan. Mum was 14 at the time, and by all accounts (well, hers at least) an innocent of the first order. She hadn't been expecting anything out of the ordinary (she said) when, going into her mother's bedroom to say goodbye before school, she was told to look in the cot beside the bed.

She looked. There was a head the size of a coconut. 'Very nice,' she said, dismissively, and started to leave. 'You could look at the other end,' said her mother. So she did. There was another one, exactly like the first. She had twin brothers!

Now that *was* interesting. Satisfying her curiosity, however, made her late for school. This was a serious offence, but Mum thought that for once she had the perfect excuse. 'My mother had twin boys last night!' she told her forbidding headmistress. But twins in those days were unusual and her headmistress didn't believe her. The outrage in Mum's voice at the injustice of being kept in after school was the climax of the story.

Mum's Alzheimer's was quite advanced before she lost her story-telling ability. At first the stories just got more outrageous. Then they started to blur into each other. The story about the twins' birth, for example, would be merged with a story about being so late for school she forgot to put on her tunic and was made to wear a bright green science overall in which she stood out like a sore thumb.

Then it was as if the telling of a story would stand, for her, as a reminder of the story, so the minute she finished it she'd start it again. I remember a particularly embarrassing lunchtime with friends at which she told the story of the twins' birth about four times, then started it another 20 times before being cut off by me saying, 'You've just told that one.'

Mum had (and has) good antennae for when she is behaving inappropriately. I fear I must have said 'You've just told that one' often enough for it to have inhibited her. But it wasn't entirely me. She had started to lose the thread of the stories. She'd start one, then get lost in it, either tailing off into embarrassed silence or making it up as she went along, so the whole was senseless. One day she just stopped.

The world is a sadder place.

> Online shopping can be a real boon. Use it both if you are caring from a distance and if you are caring at home. Why do something you needn't do? (Unless, of course, you enjoy it!) If you're not computer-literate consider using the organization Whateverage to acquire this useful skill (see the Resources chapter, pages 275–84).

Retirement

Mum didn't retire until she was 74. She enjoyed her job too much (she worked as an examiner in spoken English, travelling all over Europe to examine people taking tests in spoken English). But when she retired she retired from everything. Including housework.

She was never into housework. Or cooking. Each week she would bake a lot of apples, a dish of steak and kidney and a huge sheet of pastry. Every night she would give Dad a dollop of steak and kidney topped with a square of pastry smeared with mustard, followed by a dollop of apple topped with another square of pastry, sprinkled with sugar. This suited Dad fine. For my brother and me she would do something similar with mince and peas. It was fine by us, too.

This regime continued for Dad after Mum retired. But though Mum always kept the house tidy, the housework largely stopped. Washing up in particular became a desultory affair, involving little more than passing everything under a cold tap.

Oddly enough, though, Mum always ironed. She ironed handkerchiefs, sheets, even Dad's underpants. This wasn't desultory: everything was ironed within an inch of its life. She even taught ironing to the Girl Guides for their housework badge. This continued long after the Alzheimer's was diagnosed and she was quite proud of it.

Before she moved in I thought seriously about which jobs she could do. Everyone needs to feel useful, and I was determined that Mum wouldn't feel a burden. I could ensure that, I thought, by making sure she pulled her weight in the house.

Clearly I wasn't going to let her wash up. But she could dry up, I decided. She could also prepare vegetables. And, of course, she could iron.

Implementing this, though, wasn't easy. I was used to doing things for myself. I *like* doing things for myself. Also I quickly found that I could get away from Mum by doing something in the kitchen: her constant desire to talk can be wearing. So I found myself saying 'No' every time she asked to help.

Over the years, though, I have started to live up to my good intentions. Mum and I now end the evening by companionably doing the dishes. Often we sing raucously – 'Run Rabbit! Run Rabbit! Run, run, run' is a current favourite but we're pretty good at 'Kiss Me Goodnight Sergeant Major' and 'Don't Sit Under the Apple Tree'.

But with the ironing I really win. I have to set up the ironing board, of course, and the iron. I also have to make sure Mum doesn't leave the iron face-down. As she deteriorates, of course, the ironing is becoming increasingly erratic. But hey! Before, I hardly ironed anything. Now even my knickers are ironed!

> Mum loved being allowed – or even expected – to help.
> Maybe your piglet will, too? It's worth the mess they'll
> make. Maybe they can peg out washing, help polish the car,
> make beds, dry up, set the table and collect newspapers.
> You might even try them on the ironing.

Garden

Mum and I get on very well. But we always fall out in the garden.

I adore gardening and love to wander around in the garden, especially in the morning. I enjoy the spiders' webs sparkling in the dew, the swelling of the new buds, the overnight spurt of the new seedlings, and the smell of tomatoes in the greenhouse. I often find myself, in dressing gown and wellingtons, mucking out the compost heap at 10 a.m.

It's in the genes. My grandmother's garden was on the Beautiful Gardens of Britain calendar. Apparently (she died when I was 5) she spent every waking moment in the garden and showed every sign of liking her garden more than her children. My father, too, was a keen gardener. When I think of him it is always with his trousers tucked into his wellington boots, and a hoe over his shoulder. His constant refrain was that when he died we should throw him in the compost heap. I think he meant it.

When Dad had to go into a home because Mum couldn't look after him any more (he had stroke-induced dementia), Mum developed an interest in the garden. She would enthuse about walking around it, and spend hours weeding the lawn. God help me – I encouraged this. It kept her fit and out of mischief. I knew that she was merely pulling out the visible part of the weed, leaving the root untouched, but it didn't bother me (not my lawn, you see).

But when she moved in it *was* my lawn and it drove me completely wild. It also drove me wild that she kept pulling out what she called 'deaderies', oblivious to the fact that many plants look dead during their dormant period. I lost several clematis this way, and once spent the morning planting sweet peas, only to come down from my shower to find that Mum had pulled them all up.

Murder was nearly done that day.

Shouting at someone with Alzheimer's is no fun. Not only do you feel the anger that prompts the shouting, you also feel the guilt of knowing that the person has forgotten whatever it is they did in the first place. All the books tell you not to get angry with a demented person. The books point out that it is not them but the illness, that they can't learn from it, and that it makes everyone feel bad.

But they don't tell you *how* not to get angry with someone who has just destroyed the plants you have been nurturing for months. Nor do they mention the relief that shouting brings.

I sometimes think that people forget that Mum's feelings are not the only feelings around here.

> I never entirely solved the garden problem. But I did learn that if I sat Mum down in a chair near to where I was working, she would happily sort unopened seed packets into piles. It is amazing the different numbers of ways seed packets can be sorted. People with dementia often like to sort things: wools, books, postcards ...

A Free Agent

Mum has just spent five days with my younger brother. I have had a brilliant time, and she is full of the joys of Spring. This is partly because she doesn't know what her hair looks like. It certainly needed cutting, but I think my brother must have done it with a knife and fork.

The visit was triggered by our recent experience of respite care. This so traumatized Mum (and me) that I can't yet write about it (and shouldn't whilst our complaint goes through).

But silver clouds and all that: both my brothers now say they will look after Mum occasionally whilst I have a break.

Whoopee!

For Mum there can be few things better than staying with one of her sons. She absolutely *adores* them. She loves me and my sister, too, but we are simply not on the map when it comes to how she feels for her boys. (Yes, I do occasionally spit with the unfairness of it.)

I am (slightly) ashamed to admit to a small frisson of spiteful pleasure when she clearly isn't sure who they are. She goes along with my telling her this strange man is her son, but I don't think she really believes me. Sometimes, though, her emotional memory surfaces. When my younger brother was here last she threw her arms around his neck saying, 'I don't know who you are but I know I love you!'

But whoever she thinks he is, she had a great time with him. And I have been pretending to be a free agent.

Can you believe I spent the first day scrubbing and polishing the house? Sad or what?

But it enabled me to make the house my own. I put away all Mum's accoutrements, her trinkets and the mawkish pictures of dogs and tigers that she collects. I also played Bach and Cat Stevens at full volume (oh the bliss of not having Mum ask me to 'turn off that dreadful noise!').

The second day I spent in the garden, thinning out the cosmos and foxgloves and tying in the sweet peas. Fantastic to do this without constantly having to find jobs for Mum, or prevent her from 'weeding'.

But it wasn't all domestic bliss – I had a friend to stay, cooked supper for another, and had lunch and dinner out several times. I also watched several DVDs without having to respond every minute to Mum's off-the-wall questions: 'Is he her father?' she'll ask, as the hero and heroine finally fall into each other's arms.

It is lovely to discover I am still good at being a free agent. I revelled in the pretence of irresponsibility, and am eagerly awaiting my next opportunity.

> Age Concern (now Age UK) provided Mum with a regular podiatry service. We had to buy an inexpensive 'kit', then every six weeks Julie would turn up, cut Mum's toenails, wash and check her feet then give her a lavender foot massage. Mum was in seventh heaven! It cost £3.50 a time (in 2007).

Saints

Few would choose to care for an elderly person with dementia: total responsibility, no spontaneity, the constant need to be kind despite extreme, albeit unintentional, provocation, not to mention the cooking, cleaning, washing ...

That this is the case is obvious from people's reaction to hearing you are a carer: 'How awful!' they say, 'It must be dreadful, I simply couldn't do it.'

I am never sure how I feel about this. How would you feel about someone telling you they think your life is dreadful? But then they continue: 'You must be a complete saint.' In telling me they think my life must be dreadful, people are actually intending to place me firmly on the moral high ground. This is not without its pleasant aspects (I am ashamed to admit).

It is codswallop nevertheless. I am no saint, but merely a person who, faced with a number of dreadful options, chose the least dreadful. Maybe there are people who choose to become carers even though other, less distressing choices are available. If so, these people really are saints. But most carers, I bet, are more like me.

When Mum was diagnosed I considered buying the house next door to mine for Mum to live in. But Mum's consultant said that once she moved from the home she'd lived in for 25 years she wouldn't be able to operate independently: she would have to be cared for.

I then set out to visit a few homes. I was under the false impression that a diagnosis of Alzheimer's restricts your choice of homes, so I visited only the ones for those with dementia. I found them completely horrifying, which is not really fair as some of them do a good job in very distressing circumstances. But Mum was so far from being ready for such a place that it was completely unthinkable. It was only then that I started to consider the possibility of her moving in with me.

This quickly became the only option. Send her to a place in which she couldn't help but lose her wonderful spirit, or personally try to make the end of her life as good as she'd made the beginning of mine? What would you have done? If I had sent her to a home at that point I wouldn't have been able to live with myself.

Anyone who has ever loved another person knows that fortune thereby has a hostage. However much you feel you have life taped, if this person becomes incapable of caring for themselves, you are either going to have to care for them, or find yourself constantly questioning your own integrity for not doing so.

Anyone who says they couldn't do it might find out one day that they're wrong – perhaps they too are saints-in-waiting.

For a while Mum had weekly visits from a 'befriender' from AgeUK. Claire would sometimes whisk Mum away for a country drive ('Yes, you can keep your slippers on, we won't be getting out of the car'), other times she'd sit and chat or walk around the garden with Mum. It gave me welcome breathing space. Check your local AgeUK to see if they offer such a service.

Mum and Medication

Mum takes a cocktail of pills each morning. They are mainly vitamin pills. But they include Aricept [generic name donepezil]. This is supposed to help with cognitive impairment in the early to middle stages of dementia.

Before Mum lived with me this medication caused me huge anxiety. I would ring Mum every morning to see if she had taken it. She'd tell me she had. Mum's chief aim, by then, was to get me off her back, not to stay as healthy as possible.

I started, therefore, to ask her to get her pill dispenser and tell me which days were still full. This scuppered her attempts to pull the wool over my eyes because she had no idea what day it was. Nevertheless I lived in a state of constant anxiety about whether or not she'd taken her pills.

I then discovered that Social Services would send someone each morning to make sure Mum took her pills. I can't tell you how grateful I was. If you're a carer you don't need me to tell you.

Each morning Lynne or Anita would come along, give Mum her pills and, wherever possible, they'd stay for a chat. They were lovely people. I'm sure they were too busy for a chat, but it meant so much to Mum. Their supervision of the pill-taking meant so much to me. For the first time I felt Mum's care wasn't my sole responsibility.

Aricept has recently been in the news [2007]. NICE, the National Institute for Health and Clinical Excellence, has decided to stop funding it. They believe there is not enough evidence that the benefits, to the demented person, outweigh the cost of the pill to the nation.

Hm. Do you think they factored in the benefits to the carers?

I have to admit that I can't be certain about the cost-benefit analysis. I *think* Aricept helps Mum (and therefore me). But my only evidence for this is that when, a few years ago and before

Mum lived with me, I noticed Mum's confusion getting worse, I spoke to her consultant about increasing the Aricept. The consultant agreed. Six weeks later I'm pretty sure that Mum's confusion was less noticeable.

I can quite see that 'pretty sure' is not exactly scientific. Neither, come to that, is 'less noticeable'. If NICE tells me that the evidence is missing I suppose I must accept it.

Medical science gallops forward so fast, every new advance putting another million people on the waiting list. The cost of treating all these people must be humungous. The public purse is, of necessity, finite. Hard decisions can't be avoided. But if they didn't factor in the effect on carers we should take to the barricades.

> Social Services required me to buy a key safe [designed to store keys outside for convenience or emergency access] so that Lynne and Anita could get in even if Mum was still in bed. Even I wasn't allowed to know the combination. This infuriated me at the time. But had there been a lapse in security, this would have protected everyone from liability.

Methuselah

What a terrible night! Mum was up and down like a yo-yo until 6 a.m., when she sank into a contented but noisy sleep.

Of course that was the point at which I had to get up.

It was the cat's fault. Fatcat usually sleeps on Mum's bed, but last night she curled up beneath it. Soon after we went to bed I could hear Mum 'puss, puss, puss'-ing. Usually the cat complies fairly quickly and peace reigns. But this time it went on and on. Then I heard Mum get up and put on her light. So up I got to investigate.

I found Mum on her hands and knees asking the cat why she wouldn't come to bed. The cat had found herself a spot just out of Mum's reach and, from her lazy gaze, I could tell she had no intention of moving. I tried to tempt her out, but Fatcat and I don't see eye to eye, and if Mum couldn't move her then I wasn't going to be able to.

So I turned my persuasive skills to Mum, getting her to go back to bed on the grounds that Fatcat would join her later.

But 20 minutes later the 'puss, puss, puss'-ing started again, followed by the creaking of the bed and the flooding of the landing with light. Up I got again, and through the same routine. This happened several times and I got pretty exasperated. 'It's 1 o'clock in the morning!' I groaned. 'Is it?' she said 'I was just looking for the cat.' 'The cat doesn't want to come to bed', I snarled, 'leave the poor animal alone.'

But getting exasperated is pointless – for Mum every time is the first time, so she just thinks I'm overreacting.

At this point I did actually get to sleep. Then at 3 a.m. I was startled awake by the opening of the stair gate. Leaping out of bed I found Mum, with her clothes on over her pyjamas, grumbling that she was fed up of being moved from pillar to post and was going home.

Eh?

Goodness knows what brought that on, but an hour later the same thing happened, except that Mum had actually started to negotiate the stairs. The stair gate, of course, is supposed to stop her from going downstairs. But she's a wily old bird and extremely determined. Thankfully this doesn't happen very often, though every night we're up at least once or twice.

Today, though, I feel like Methuselah's grandmother while Mum, when I got her up for day care, seemed her usual sprightly self.

Tonight no doubt she'll complain, when I want to go to bed at 7 p.m., that I have no staying power.

> Have you re-thought your home since becoming a carer? If you've patched and adapted in an ad hoc manner as your piglet deteriorated you might be unaware of the hugely useful adaptations that could be made as the result of a proper risk- and need-assessment. They could transform your life. Social Services will arrange a risk-assessment and can often pay for smaller changes.

Deafness

Mum is going deaf. It is maddening.

An uncharitable response, you might think, but you try it. The worst times are when I utter a minor pleasantry, or offer a scrap of unnecessary information, just to make her feel we're conversing. Last night, for example, I said something about Fatcat looking comfortable as I manoeuvred round her on the way upstairs (she – Fatcat that is – likes to spread herself out on the corner stair).

'What?' said Mum. 'Oh b*****' I thought to myself. 'What did you say?' she repeated. 'Old Fatcat looks comfortable' I yelled, knowing that as I was halfway upstairs it would be useless.

You're probably thinking: why don't you just tell her again when you come down? The answer is that if, by the third time of asking, Mum still hasn't heard she'll start heaving herself out of the sofa to find me so she doesn't miss anything.

This creates such a palaver I can't bear it. For a start, my sofas were not bought with 87-year-old ladies in mind. I like to sink into a sofa, and before Mum arrived these were perfect. They are far from perfect now. As soon as I hear the grunt that precedes the heaving I'll try almost anything to stop the process ('Don't worry, Mum, I'll bring it for you,' 'Please don't get up Mum, I'll get it.').

So there I am halfway up the stairs, and I hear the grunt. Immediately I reverse and start running down, screeching 'I only said Fatcat was looking comfortable. Don't get up!'

Too late. Mum is up, surrounded by the pages of her newspaper (which she'll put back upside-down and in the wrong order), her spectacles askew, trailing her blanket, and looking anxious. She has already forgotten why she was getting up, and now I am telling her to sit down again. Life is very confusing.

A while ago I agreed to a free hearing test for Mum. The man arrived, set up his kit and conducted the test, despite Mum's protests that I was just making a fuss, there's nothing wrong with her hearing.

When he showed her the results (Surprise! A clear deficit), she dismissed them, insisting that I had not been speaking clearly enough.

Outrageous! She taught me to speak herself, and as befits a senior examiner in spoken English, she did a good job (though I say so myself).

So we bought a hearing aid. But has she ever worn it? Of course not. It lives in a drawer, and we have reverted to my having to repeat everything while she admonishes me for whispering.

Oh, well, it was worth a try …

> Your piglet will reach a point where getting them a hearing aid is pointless. As they don't remember what it is or what it is for, they'll just keep removing it. Either make sure they get an aid before this point, or learn to speak LOUDLY AND CLEARLY.

Dream

This week I'd like you to close your eyes, bring your piglet and come with me on an imaginary journey. We're going to a place where the care system *works*.

This is a place where substitute care is available in the *evenings* (let's go to the cinema!) and *on Sunday* (come for lunch!), not just from 10–3 on weekdays.

Here professional carers and special buses *arrive on time*: you will never again weep as your train leaves without you or you miss the first half-hour of the class.

If you fall under a bus, the heating breaks down, your piglet falls or your train is delayed, you will be able to ring a magic telephone number, manned 24/7, and *everything will be dealt with*. Within minutes an ambulance (or plumber) will have been called, your neighbour will be at your door and/or your sister's car will be out. You'll be able to concentrate on the crisis knowing that help is coming.

Here the expense of caring is acknowledged in free travel for you and your piglet, and in discounts on utilities and Council tax. Places of entertainment offer carers' discounts and regularly put on piglet-friendly shows.

Shopping centres have places where piglets can be left for an hour or two. Your piglet loves these places and is *reluctant to leave*! No reason, therefore, *not* to have a coffee and read the paper when the shopping's done.

In this place your medical records and those of your piglet have large, red, *accurate* notes saying you are their carer. These notes are *read* and *acted on*. So your appointment will be convenient and you will not be kept waiting. A specialist carer-supporter will keep your piglet happy while you go to the loo, and brief the doctor. You will smile serenely (!) as your piglet insists that they take no medication: no need for frantic semaphores behind their head.

In this place you are not only 'entitled to' respite care, you *get* it. What's more, it's available whenever you need (or want) it. Your piglet can go for one night (you *can* go to the ball), a weekend (you'll make the wedding), or mid-week (catch up with that paperwork. Have a rest).

And when they come back from respite they are – wait for it – healthy and cheerful. They don't have to be scrubbed, comforted or rehydrated. You will not need to take them to the dentist (to replace their lost teeth), the department store (to replace their lost underwear), or the doctor's (to get rid of that nasty urinary infection).

Oho! That woke you up, didn't it? Yes, sorry, perhaps that was a step too far. But wasn't it a lovely dream?

> I used to represent carers on Social Services committees. But poor briefing and prolific use of jargon and acronyms made it impossible to make a useful contribution consistently with my available time and energy. I gave up. Are you made of sterner stuff? Contact Social Services and give it a go.

Dress Sense

In the middle of yesterday's morning dash, I found Mum sitting on her bed, holding a sock in each hand, and looking puzzled.

'What's wrong?' I asked.

'I've only got two socks' she replied.

Getting Mum dressed gets harder by the day. We have just given up on tights. All of a sudden she forgot how to put them on. One day she was unrolling them onto her legs as if it were second nature, the next she was putting her foot in and trying to pull them up. As every woman reader will know, this does not work, and she was getting very frustrated.

At first I tried to put them on for her but life is too short for such shenanigans – socks it'll be from now on.

It's such a shame because Mum used to have a tremendous sense of style. She was tall and willowy slim, with legs to die for. She bought classic clothes and wore them well: a picture of elegance. I have a picture of Mum at 17 looking every inch a young Catherine Zeta-Jones.

She particularly enjoyed wearing colours, and she chose them well. I used to love dressing up in one of her old cocktail dresses, a swirling kaleidoscope of shimmering silk, still smelling faintly of her perfume.

It might even be said that she was vain – her sister, a no-nonsense farmer's wife, once said sniffily to me: 'Your mother is one of those women whose shoes have to match her bag.' So they did: Mum would no more go out in an unmatched outfit than without her purse.

But Mum has lost her sense of style. I now choose her clothes. I give her the illusion of choice by offering her alternatives, but I shamelessly exploit the fact she'll always choose the last offered item to make sure she is dressed reasonably well.

If I didn't she would dress as she dressed the other day when she got up early and made her own choices: blue trousers tucked into long black socks, a leopard print top over a dark red blouse, and a pair of large peacock blue enamel earrings.

It hurts me as much to see her like this as it must have hurt her to put up with the tie-dye granddad shirts and Indian headbands of my teenage years.

But it's not all bad. Mum's ritual, before going out, was always to twirl for me so I could exclaim on her beauty. Now, whenever I go out, I twirl for her, and am sent on my way with her coos about *my* beauty ringing in my ears.

Few more satisfying ways to start an evening!

The fact your piglet will always choose the last mentioned item in any list means it is always possible to offer them a choice consistently while nudging them in a particular direction. If, like me, you are a control freak who believes in autonomy for piglets, this is very satisfying.

Marriage

Mum always bemoaned the fact she'd never had a wedding dress. But she adored having eloped on Dad's motorbike.

They met in Windsor Great Park. She was walking her 3-year-old twin brothers and lolloping red setter. He and his brother were boating on the lake. Supervising the twins was not, at 17, a priority. But at least she panicked on realizing they were gone.

Searching everywhere, she finally spotted them in a boat in the middle of the lake with two strangers. With the fury of relief she stood on the bank screaming 'How *dare* you? Bring them back *right now*.'

Now Dad takes up the story. The young men had been accosted by the twins, fascinated by their boat and insisting on a ride. Without a thought in their heads, the boys decided to give the twins a treat.

When they became aware of the virago on the bank, they felt chastened and hurried back. Dad, as they approached, saw the woman he would marry. It was, he said, as simple as that: he loved her from the moment he saw her.

The same could not be said of her. As soon as the twins scrambled out of the boat she swept them off with a haughty toss of her ponytail.

But my dad was nothing if not tenacious. He knocked on doors asking for a family with a girl of about 17, twin boys of 3 and a red setter until he found her. Answering the door to his knock, my horrified Mum hissed 'Go away!' and slammed the door in his face.

He persisted and, in the teeth of her parents' opposition (their money was on the boy next door), he won her. She claimed she was never sure whether it was her parents' stubbornness or the looming war that did the trick.

They married in a small registry office ceremony during which she lied about her age and met her mother-in-law for the first time (*that* wasn't love at first sight, either). It was 2nd November 1939.

Their marriage wasn't made in heaven. But it worked. They weathered the war, brought up four children and managed their chalk-and-cheese personalities. He continued to adore her. She treated him abominably. But when a stroke left him with dementia her love for him manifested itself in a fierce determination to care for him.

When he died they had been married for 61 years and 19 days. Mum was, herself, by then in the grip of Alzheimer's. Now her memory is completely shot. But mention Dad and she will unfailingly smile happily and say, 'He was a lovely man, wasn't he?'

I reckon that's a pretty good epitaph, don't you?

> If your piglet's long-term memory is still OK go through their old photographs with them, identifying the people portrayed – together, if possible, with details of the scene. Write these details on the back. This can be fun. If your piglet's long-term memory is shot, don't do this: it will upset them.

Shopping

When Dad retired he took over the shopping. He would snip coupons out of the local newspapers, collect every voucher going and spend hours comparing prices. Then he would plot his route around the shops so he didn't waste shoe leather.

He would set off, shopping bag in hand, hat on head and a determined expression on his face. On his return he would deliver a smug commentary on the money he had saved and the bargains he had made.

Anyone else would have clocked him. But Mum was only too happy to have the shopping done. After all, she'd been doing it herself for 40-odd years. Putting up with his smugness was reasonable compensation, she thought, for not having to do it any more.

For all their married life Mum and Dad kept separate accounts. They had monthly reckonings to see who owed what to whom. One would solemnly hand the other the twopence ha'penny owed, and on they would go. Mum insisted on this – she believed strongly in female independence and always kept a 'running-away fund' (and advised her daughters to do likewise).

Both Mum and Dad kept very full accounts of their expenditure. I have them all, and interesting reading they make. On Tuesday 20th October 1961 Mum's shopping list starts with 15 milk tokens and includes half a pound of lard, half a pound of butter, four pounds of granulated sugar, two bags of potatoes, Typhoo tea and 10 Senior Service cigarettes.

This gives an accurate reflection of their diet: Dad was a great believer in 'oiling the joints' with plenty of fat, and his cup of tea was more sugar than tea. He also smoked 60 cigarettes a day (the 10 Senior Service were probably for Mum). How he lived to 84 is a mystery. Maybe it was the sulphur tablets he insisted on taking in Spring.

The bill for this particular shopping list came to £2, 11 shillings and 5½ d. Mum would have been to the Co-op and she would have made sure she got her Green Shield stamps and Co-op coupons. Sometimes she sent me, and woe betide me if I forgot the stamps. The shop assistants, kindly middle-aged women, would give me a ha'penny chew for helping Mummy. I was secretly in love with the butcher.

Mum no longer worries about money. Her accounts tail off in 1997. The Alzheimer's was diagnosed in 1999. Sometimes, out shopping, she'll search herself for money to buy me flowers or chocolate. She loves to be told that, like the Queen, she never carries money.

I notice, though, that in her bedside chest there is a collection of coins knotted in a handkerchief. Alzheimer's or not, she still has her running-away fund!

I thought it important, while Mum's dementia was reasonably mild, to make sure she had money to spend on things that took her fancy. Mum had become a magpie, adoring anything that sparkled or glittered. She loved to look around charity shops and invariably bought something that gave her pleasure.

Teeth

It is a source of pride for my mum that, at 87, she still has a lot of her own teeth.

Actually she doesn't have half as many as she thinks she has. There was a time when every time I looked at her there was another one missing. We spent so much time at the dentist that he was considering charging us rent.

The fact is that if you give up cleaning your teeth they will fall out. And Mum gave up cleaning her teeth soon after the Alzheimer's was diagnosed.

Of course she would (and does) deny this strenuously: 'How could I forget to clean my teeth?' she'll ask in a voice of outrage, or 'I can forget a lot of things but certainly *not* my teeth!'

Hm. When she moved in with me I insisted she brush her teeth twice a day. Mum became a shameless liar. Despite conclusive evidence to the contrary (a toothbrush still fully charged with toothpaste), she would insist she had done them. But Mum's a lousy liar (a memory, after all, is the *sine qua non* of a successful liar) and we were constantly at war over her teeth.

But all this vigilance meant her teeth stopped falling out. Now if at bedtime she sneaks under the covers before she's done her teeth, I only have to say 'teeth!' for her to heave herself up again, grumbling all the while.

She has, though, lost enough teeth to have to wear a denture. During Mum's recent debacle with respite care, this denture was lost.

Like most people without teeth, Mum looked pitiful. Her face caved in and her mouth became pinched. She looked like the Wicked Witch of the West.

Because Mum wasn't conscious of the lack, however, others soon forgot. She would smile as often and as widely as usual, and after the initial recoil people quickly adapted. Indeed, I wondered whether I mightn't be able to scrub 'getting Mum new dentures' off my 'to do' list.

But teeth are rather useful. Especially for eating. I was having to cut everything into tiny pieces for her, a job far more onerous then putting dentures into Steradent twice a day.

In the end, though, it is a dignity matter. Mum without her teeth was somehow a lesser person. When she was interacting with others this was less obvious, but when she was reading the paper or watching television she seemed to have become a stereotypical old woman.

I refuse to let Mum become a stereotypical old woman.

So we renewed our acquaintance with the dentist. Two weeks ago her new dentures arrived, twice a day I wield the Steradent, and Mum is a person again.

Two weeks after I first wrote this blog entry, Mum lost her new teeth. £450 worth. I decided it simply wasn't worth the bother any more and resigned myself to cutting her food up. I don't think she ever noticed the lack.

Coughing

Last month was terrible. I had been overdoing it ('So what else is new?' I hear friends ask). Anyway, after five cold-free years I caught a string of coughs and colds that laid me really low.

No one likes being ill, but for a carer it is the pits. I sat forlornly in a chair, head throbbing, longing for someone to offer me a cup of tea. Instead not only did I have to make my own tea, I also had to carry on with everything else, including washing, dressing, feeding, watering and amusing Mum.

Periodically I tried to get sympathy from Mum. Sometimes she'd give me a hug and ask if she could do anything. But to be honest Mum never was a sympathizer. 'Well, never mind,' she'd say briskly, 'it'll soon disappear.' Or worse: 'Just don't give it to me!'

As for her making me tea – well, last time I got a cup of cold water into which she had stirred a spoonful of coffee grounds and half a carton of strawberry yoghurt. (When we had builders in I adored their attempts to deal with Mum's offerings.) When Mum makes tea not only do I get no tea, I also get to deal with the fallout from Mum's making it.

It's not so bad when she goes to day care. Then I can crawl back to bed and make up some cough-destroyed sleep. But first I have to get Mum up, wash her, dress her, give Mum and the cats their breakfast and wait for the special bus (which can be half an hour late). If I left her sleeping I'd still have to get up to cancel the bus and ring the day care centre. Then it's sod's law that Mum would get up an hour later and I'd have to keep her amused for the whole day.

Obviously if it were a real emergency I would ring friends or family and beg for help. But a cough is not a real emergency. I feel bad about asking friends to look after Mum when they all have jobs and responsibilities of their own. My family all live quite far away (and again have their own responsibilities).

No, what's needed is a rota of professional 'supply carers' like the teachers who go into schools when teachers are ill. So from her sickbed a carer could ring a number, croak out the problem, and someone would swoop in like a super-hero and just deal with it.

Yeah. Right.

But my cough is better (thank you for asking). Now I only have to deal with the fact that Mum caught it.

Actually that idea about supply carers is a good one, isn't it? My Council was forever promising carers a special emergency number (it never happened). If they ever actually do it, this could be one of the services offered. With all the agencies around it shouldn't be too hard to organize. Suggest it to your Council.

Crashing Cars in the Sun

The sun is finally shining. There are squeals of laughter coming from the garden. Mum is playing with Andrej, Anita's two-year-old son.

Andrej has lined up his dinky cars and he's rolling them down the table one by one, accompanied by loud *brrmming* noises. Mum is catching them as they come and crashing them into the next with the same *brrmming* noises. Both are cackling gleefully at every crash.

They have been doing this for two hours and neither is showing sign of losing interest. Mum's boredom is temporarily banished and Andrej is manfully putting up with being smothered with kisses every few minutes.

I have noticed often that the very young – pre-school children – are completely accepting of the very old. They don't see them as odd, musty and decrepit, they just see someone who has the time and patience endlessly to play with them.

Here are people who are not constantly rushed. People who are happy to watch worms, read and re-read stories and answer questions. People who are not constantly nagging you to do something you don't want to do. What's not to like?

As for the very old, well, if Mum is representative, they *adore* the young. Andrej only has to walk through the door, yelling endearingly as he does: 'Lesley, Lesley, where's Lesley?' for her to drop ten years. Mum comes alive in Andrej's company.

The very young are – in the jargon – a resource for the very old, and vice versa. They are a resource, furthermore, that costs nothing. They entertain each other and provide exactly what the other needs.

Yet you'd almost think there was a policy to keep them apart. Do you know any nursing homes attached to crèches? Day care centres in nurseries? Exactly. We treat the care of these two groups of people completely separately. But wouldn't it enhance the lives of both groups if they were cared for together?

I know older people sometimes go into schools to talk about their experiences of the war, or of growing up in a different era. I hear heart-warming tales of children open-mouthed with wonder, and older people basking in their interest. I have also heard of schoolchildren visiting the elderly and recording their memories.

Wonderful! But it doesn't go far enough. When I am Prime Minister I shall combine nurseries and day care centres. No residential home will be without a crèche. The very young and the very old will flourish as a result of spending time together.

Obviously there'd have to be safeguards. We don't want elderly people tripping over building bricks, or babies being dropped as supper is announced. But where there's a will …

> Mum loved to be taken to children's playgrounds. She'd
> watch them play for hours. She also liked a sneaky go on
> the swings or the roundabout. I have heard they are setting
> up activity parks for elderly people. What an excellent idea.
> Let's have more. Perhaps there's one near you?

Qualifications

Mum went to secretarial college at 17. There wasn't much option. She wanted to be a nurse but her parents wouldn't consider it. Both her brothers went to university but that was deemed unsuitable for girls. So secretarial college it was.

Being a secretary wasn't her thing. She did it until I was born, probably because the war and two children stopped her from working much. But when I came along she had had enough of being a mother and a secretary. She set out to get some qualifications.

She decided to teach Spoken English. This involved several years of part-time study. Maive, a friend of Mum's, tells me that Mum took to study like a duck to water. She particularly recalls my being balanced on Mum's hip whilst Mum, oblivious to my screams, stirred a sauce and read from a book perched on the work surface.

I have Mum's public speaking medals – all distinctions and merits, each one making her more determined to continue. Once qualified, she worked for the English Speaking Board. She would regale us with stories of the youngsters she examined and the props they used in their talks. These once included a live snake.

But still Mum wanted more intellectual stimulation. At 65 she started an Open University course.

She absolutely *adored* it and became an OU groupie – TMA [tutor-marked assignment] this, CMA [computer-marked assignment] that, tutorials and summer schools were all grist to her mill. She wasn't seen for hours when she had an essay deadline, and during her exams she disappeared for days.

Eventually, yearning to study full-time, she went to finish her degree at a nearby university. She was by far the oldest student. The others treated her as a mascot. Her university was notoriously left-wing and my instinctively liberal democrat Mum became a slogan-spouting leftie.

One day the telephone rang. The caller said: 'This is Lesley Talbot.' 'Odd,' I thought, but before I could say anything, she said 'Lesley Talbot BA.' 'Aha,' I thought. Then she said: 'Lesley Talbot BA, UPPER SECOND CLASS!!!'

I whooped, she whooped, and the words started tumbling out: 'I haven't felt like this' she said, 'since Christopher was a baby. Daddy was on leave, it was a beautiful summer's day and we took some bread and some precious butter to the hills and had a picnic. We were in love with each other and with our baby. I couldn't believe how wonderful the world was. I feel like that now.'

She was 70 years old. It was 1989, the year of her 50th wedding anniversary. I was so proud of her. It was only ten years later that she was diagnosed with Alzheimer's.

Makes every minute seem precious, doesn't it?

> I have a photograph of Mum at her graduation. Wearing cap and gown and clutching her certificate, she has a beatific smile on her face. I adore the photograph. Mum used to love being talked through that photograph, together with her medals and certificates. Is there a photographic record of something of which your piglet was hugely proud?

Phoebe

Yesterday Hubert and Phoebe came to tea. Phoebe is Mum's special friend from Willows, her day care centre. She has vascular dementia and is a complete delight.

Most of the time, like Mum, Phoebe is away with the fairies. But she obviously enjoys it there. She has a lovely smile, and responds enthusiastically to everything one says. At least, she does when she hears it.

'Would you like a scone?' I asked Phoebe. Nothing. 'Marianne asked you if you'd like a scone,' says Hubert. 'A scone?' says Phoebe, 'A scone! I'd love a scone, how absolutely marvellous, a scone! Oh yes please.'

Mum clearly feels responsible for Phoebe when they're on Mum's territory. She buttered Phoebe's scone (getting butter *everywhere*), asked if she'd like another cup of tea, and told her to drink up if she wanted another.

But just when it was beginning to feel like a vicar's tea party, Mum gave Phoebe a great smacking kiss, and told her she was beautiful. Phoebe, wreathed in smiles, returned the compliment and they beamed at each other in adoration.

Then Fatcat waddled out. 'Oh!' said Phoebe, 'Pussycat, pussycat where have you been?' she sang energetically. 'I've been to London to see the Queen' warbled Mum. They looked at each other, giggled, and started again. Neither could remember any more words, but they simply made them up, laughing delightedly at themselves. Impossible not to feel like a fond parent.

I felt the same suggesting that Mum show Phoebe the garden, so Hubert and I could talk. 'Ooooh,' said Phoebe, 'I'd *love* to see the garden. Such a beautiful garden, oh yes please.' Off they went hand in hand like two little girls, heads together, oohing and ahhing. Then, collapsing onto the swing seat, they started hooting like owls.

So they were happy. And Hubert and I were able to talk. Yesterday we found ourselves laughing at the situations we get into trying to anticipate disaster in respect of someone whose behaviour is informed by 87 years' worth of habit.

If I leave the table during a meal, for example, Mum will

immediately start clearing plates, irrespective of the fact people have only just started and food is cascading everywhere. Or she will hang out the washing (which is great) only to take it all in again 2 minutes later when I am not looking. Phoebe is the same.

But they're also the same in their life-enhancing qualities and, when the time comes for Hubert and Phoebe to leave, it is a joy to watch Mum and Phoebe blow kisses to each other until the car is out of sight.

Two seconds later Mum has forgotten Phoebe was even there.

> Phoebe, as I write, is in great health. She walks every day and has an unbelievable appetite. Naturally she doesn't remember Mum. I flatter myself that she has some memory of me when I go round occasionally to sit with her. Her life-enhancing qualities are intact despite her now very severe dementia.

Revenge

When Mum first came to live with me we went to church every Sunday. It was a lovely church, 1,000 years old and surrounded by ancient graves. Not quite my thing – the vicar is dead against women priests – but only 5 minutes' walk away. Mum enjoyed the fact we were doing something together.

But then she started objecting to being woken. 'Why have I got to get up?' she'd demand. 'We're going to church.' I'd say. 'Why?' she'd ask.

Good question. If she didn't want to go to church, why was I taking her? I told myself that deep down she really wanted to go.

But it's possible I was revenging myself on her for forcing my brother and me to church every Sunday. Like it or not we were scrubbed, made to dress up, be quiet and go to Sunday School.

I suspect that Mum's motive for making us go to church was at least partly revenge on her part, as Dad was virulently anti-church. He believed, he said, that a chap called 'Jesus' once existed, but he was no son of God. Anyway he hated the 'mumbo-jumbo'. I thought this was sophistication itself, and tried refusing to go to church. But Mum wasn't having it.

Dad got his own revenge when Mum went to Evensong, leaving us in his care. He let us do whatever we wanted. Our favourite game was to slide, in our socks, down the long polished dining table, propelled by a push from the other. Screaming with laughter we'd fall off the end into a pile of cushions, then go round and start again. Unperturbed by the mayhem Dad read his paper, smoked his cigarette and drank his tea.

But then a particularly good push of mine sent Richard head-first through the French windows.

There was a great deal of blood, and Richard was carted off to hospital. I thought it was his usual fuss about nothing, especially when he stayed home from school the next day. But Mum was furious. From then on we went to Evensong, too.

So revenge and church attendance are intertwined for me. But trying to drag an unwilling mother to church soon palled. First I struggled to get her out of bed. Then I struggled to get her there with her driving me batty by asking every five seconds 'How far are we going along here?' So it started to feel silly, especially as she got nothing out of the service.

These days I leave Mum asleep, and I find God in the garden. I'm sure He understands.

Your piglet may find attending church services comforting. If they were ever a church-goer, the rituals will be second nature. They might even remember the words of the prayers and the tunes of the hymns. How nice for someone with dementia to feel familiar with what is going on.

Cats

Fatcat has been the light of Mum's life for 13 years. I knew that when Mum came to live with me, therefore, Fatcat would come too.

Fatcat is not my favourite animal. When she is crossed – often, as I refuse to let Mum feed her – she glares hatred from huge golden eyes. She is too big to wash herself so has to be brushed and, despite the diet I've had her on for four years, she cannot get out of the cat-flap. On occasion, caught short, she has peed under my desk. I could cheerfully strangle her.

My sister suggested I do just that. But one look at Mum's face when Fatcat waddles in and it's obvious the blasted cat is a fixture.

When Mum is due home from day care Fatcat waits outside. As the bus arrives she heaves herself to her feet and looks intently at the gate. As Mum descends Fatcat does her party piece: she makes straight for Mum, stops and stretches out her paw, for all the world as if saying 'Where have you *been*?'

Mum simply melts. Delightedly she fusses over a loudly purring Fatcat, exclaiming 'This cat seems to know me!' or 'Look, this cat likes me!' Once inside I make tea and Mum renews her acquaintance with Fatcat who, still purring, butts her head repeatedly against Mum's legs.

Easy to see why research suggests that elderly people are healthier and happier when there are animals around.

Dad detested cats. We used to have two, a small one called Timpkins (don't ask) and a large one called Candy. They popped out of the patch pocket of Mum's tweed coat when I was 5.

Dad was horrified. But he was outvoted. He could often be heard muttering darkly about 'bloody cats'. He liked to threaten to feed the little one to the big one and eat the big one for Sunday lunch. He wasn't above giving them a sly kick. I once saw him kick Candy, whose loud squawk he immediately explained in terms of the 'bloody animal continuously getting under my feet'.

Sometimes, as Dad read his paper, one of the cats would decide his lap looked inviting. Mum would signal excitedly to us and, as the cat gathered strength for an elegant leap onto Dad's lap, we'd all watch, collapsing into giggles as Dad leapt up, knocking the startled cat to the ground and expostulating that we should choose between the cats and him because he was *not* going to put up with this any longer.

If Mum were away, though, he would feed them: 'There you are, bloody cat' he would say, 'breakfast'. Feeding Fatcat, I know just how Dad felt.

> If your piglet, like Mum, was an animal lover, you might consider taking them to a 'children's farm'. These places keep animals such as rabbits, lambs, piglets and ponies in an environment that is safe for children. Children (and others) can feed and pet the animals and watch them to their heart's content.

Party Animal

'All's fair in love and war,' Dad said smugly when explaining why he had claimed to love the theatre while courting Mum. Married in 1939, opportunities to go to the theatre were limited. It took ages for Mum to discover he'd been lying.

It wasn't just the theatre Dad disliked, it was also the cinema ('It'll be on television soon'), the opera ('dreadful noise'), dining out ('They never warm the plates'), anything that involved leaving his armchair.

So when Mum came to live with me I encouraged her to be the party animal I think she should have been.

We went to films, plays, opera and the ballet. We dined out, lunched in pubs and even went to a garden party at the Palace.

That was fun: the Queen stopped to talk only 6 feet away. Mum almost swooned with excitement.

She was touchingly appreciative: 'I do like living with you,' she'd say, leaning over to give me a kiss. Her manifest enjoyment of everything was infectious. I found myself enjoying things all the more for being with her.

But this gadding didn't last long. The first to go was the cinema. You probably don't even notice the advertisements, but they are extremely LOUD and very cOnFuSiNg. Mum flinched at every bang, and kept looking to me for reassurance.

Then the theatre became impossible. Mum responded to her inability to follow the plot by assuming there was something wrong with the play. She'd turn to me and make 'isn't this dreadful?' faces, or say loudly 'What on Earth are they talking about?' causing me to cringe with embarrassment.

The opera lasted longer. But I started to resent paying £40 for something Mum forgot immediately. I bought Mum DVDs of her favourite operas instead. She loves to sing along with *Carmen*, for example, though I have to dash in before José stabs Carmen because that won't do at all.

Now even watching television with Mum is painful. Mum constantly asks me what is going on in a way that makes it clear that she isn't even at first base. 'Are they just getting up?' she asks, as the robbers dash to their car. Throughout she'll say, 'I have no idea what is going on' or 'What's happening?' clearly certain that only she is in step.

So I have given up watching television myself. I record things to watch when she's in bed. But I never get around to watching them (not least because, exhausted, I usually go to bed when she does, even if that's at 8 p.m.).

We spend the evening reading (or in Mum's case looking at pictures) in companionable silence. I am probably all the better for it.

> When buying music for your piglet, if you go for 'songs from the Second World War' or suchlike make sure you listen before you buy: I bought a set, each disc of which started with the air-raid alarm. Why would anyone do that to someone who lived through the blitz?!

Sticker-inner

Mum may have Alzheimer's but she can still give as good as she gets. The other night was the usual rush, it was late and I was getting ratty.

I was outside trying to remember which bin to put out when, from the kitchen, she called me. 'Yes?' I yelled. But she didn't hear and called again, 'Where *are* you?!' There was nothing for it but to leave what I was doing and find out what she wanted.

'Now what?' I said testily 'I'm putting the bin out.' 'I think you should put yourself in it,' said Mum promptly.

Then there was the time when, pulling her socks off, I said 'What odd feet you've got' and she immediately riposted 'At least I haven't got a green neck' in obvious reference to the polo neck I was wearing.

I love it when she does this, not least because recently she has been losing her grip on language.

She loses her words a lot. Sometimes she gives up in frustration. But at other times she can be delightfully inventive. The television becomes the 'noise box', the newspaper the 'word thing', a knife the 'sticker-inner' (interestingly Freudian, this one).

The aptness of her inventions suggests to me that there is still an intellect in there, however difficult it is for her to express it.

This manifests itself in other ways, too. Recently she poured her coffee into her cereal and when I said (rather pathetically) 'You've just poured your coffee into your cereal' she replied, 'Yes,

I know, but they belong to each other' and ate it all quite happily.

Language was always hugely important to Mum. She used to delight in reading us the nonsense verses. In the car she would encourage us to make up stories, and compete with us to see who could make the best words from the number plates of passing cars. She'd never tell us the meaning of a word, we always had to look it up (because this was the only way to remember), and she'd constantly correct our pronunciation.

Interestingly, despite her deterioration she still gets pleasure from language. The newspaper recently had a supplement on word play. It listed a number of pairs of words that are confused with each other. Mum loved this list. 'Turbid/turgid' she'd say, 'vicious/viscous', 'specious/ spurious', each word carefully articulated. She would read it to me again and again, with no idea what it was actually about, just enjoying the sounds of the words as she uttered them.

Every hour or so, though, I have to hide the paper so I don't get the sticker-inner and stick it in 'er!

> Pinning notes up is useful in the initial stages of dementia: 'hot tap' 'switch' etc. But your piglet will pass the point of assigning meaning to written words. It's so easy to assume – wrongly – that because you attach meaning to a label, they will, too. So easy, too, for your fear to express itself in irritation towards your poor piglet. When the notes stop being useful, get rid of them.

Irritation

Last Thursday was Mum's birthday. 88 years and counting! I woke her with a raucous rendition of 'Happy Birthday to You' and told her she was 108. She groaned and said she didn't want to know.

Her cards were waiting for her at breakfast. But she couldn't work out how to use the paper knife so I had to open them. Then I had to read them to her because she kept holding them upside-down or back to front. After each one she said in a voice of amazement: 'Is it my birthday?'

She said it again when the day care people sang 'Happy Birthday' as she went to the bus, and no doubt said it several hundred times during the day. She was still saying it when she got home.

A few friends came for tea. I had cooked a chestnut and chocolate cake and we opened a bottle of champagne. Mum opened her presents, amazed to discover, at each one, that it was her birthday. (She kept adding, irritatingly: 'I didn't know' or 'No one told me.' Gggggrrr.)

The tea party became a supper party. In our small kitchen I was therefore simultaneously juggling cups, saucers and cake plates, and trying to prepare and cook an impromptu stir fry.

Fatcat, hoping I would drop something, was winding herself around my feet. Mum, wanting to help, was hovering at my elbow.

'What can I do?' she offered.

'Nothing at the moment,' I replied 'Go and entertain your guests.'

Off she wandered. But 30 seconds later there she was again. 'Is there anything I can do?'

'It's easier at the moment if I do it myself' I said. 'Go and talk to Joelle.'

Not 20 seconds later she was back 'Can I help at all?'

AAAAaaargh!

You'd think, wouldn't you, that I'd have predicted it? It's not as if it hasn't happened before. Why didn't I devise a few jobs to take her out of my way and make her feel useful? She would have been happy and I could have preened myself on my foresight.

Instead she felt in the way and I felt stressed and irritated. And guilty. Instead of making Mum happy, I had made her feel surplus to requirements. It's not even as if the things I was so intent on doing mattered: she still had no idea it was her birthday.

As far as she was concerned, a take-away would have done. Especially if I had held her hand and helped her talk to everyone while we waited for it to be delivered.

It is when I am trying my hardest to be perfect that I most show my feet of clay.

Looking back on this one makes me sad. Mum had started to lose her grip on social situations. Previously this had been very much her métier. She only felt safe, I think, when she was with familiar people. This puts an extra pressure on the carer, of course, who is the most familiar person.

Curtains

An irritating thing about people with Alzheimer's is that, until you learn a few tricks, they always get their own way. It is amazing how a total lack of memory confers the upper hand.

Every evening, for example, as the night draws in, Mum and I have the same conversation:

Mum: 'Shall I draw the curtains?'

Me: 'No, it'll be light for a couple of hours yet.'

Two minutes later:

Mum: 'Shall I draw the curtains?'

Me (louder): 'Not yet, it's still light.'

Two minutes later:

Mum: 'Shall I draw the curtains?'

Me (groaning): 'Oh go on then.'

There's no compromising with someone with Alzheimer's. Mum likes the curtains closed and cannot take on board that I prefer them open.

Then there's the bed-making. Mum makes the bed the minute she gets out of it. I like beds to air. It was a year before I realized Mum was never going to learn not to make the bed. Talk about asking for stress: she'd make the bed, then I'd unmake it and tell her (again) that I prefer it to air. She'd say 'I'll remember next time.' Huh.

This was a recipe for starting the day in a bad mood. But then I started learning a few tricks.

Nowadays Mum makes the bed and, as soon as she goes downstairs, I unmake it. Simple. Why didn't I think of it before? It was partly the stress of getting used to her living with me, and partly, I blush to admit, control freakery on my part.

It was just as simple – when I finally thought about it – to deal with the washing up problem. I hated Mum washing up (she passes things under the cold tap then immediately dries them, getting bits of food all over the tea cloth). I used to try to stop her, but then we'd have the conversation in which she'd ask why she shouldn't wash up, I'd reply she was useless at it, she'd protest she'd been washing up for hundreds of years and I'd retort that she ought to have learned how to do it properly.

But now, unless I actually *want* this conversation (believe it or not it can be fun) I let Mum wash up, then I distract her, then I do the washing up again. Properly. Works brilliantly.

Another type of trick involves simply refusing to get irritated. I can't stop Mum reading out the same bit of the newspaper 20 times, so I have learned how not to get irritated. This may sound odd, but it works. If I respond in exactly the same way every time I don't even have to listen, far less think about a reply.

Now I just have to stop myself doing this at work!

Interesting to see how smug I sometimes felt. I undoubtedly learned many tricks as I went along. But don't for one minute get the impression I had it taped. As soon as I learned one set of tricks, another of Mum's abilities would atrophy and I'd need a whole new set.

Forgiving Oneself

Mum is a wise old bird. I contemplated saying 'was', but she still has what it takes. Recently I quoted to her Marlowe's line 'Whoever loved that loved not at first sight?'

'Huh!' she snorted 'Poppycock!'

Well, I think that deals with that one.

When I was a teenager she was the perfect mum. She wasn't all over me, but she showed concern. We were once driving to church the morning after I had parted from a boyfriend. 'If you've been crying' she said 'mascara draws attention to it.' This unleashed the tears, and the story. Mum listened, comforted and stroked my bruised self-esteem.

Whenever there is a furore over gay rights I think of her take on homosexuality: 'Love' she said 'is in short enough supply. Everyone has the right to find it where they can.' I was about 15 when she said this to me. I sensed she was telling me that if I was gay this wouldn't be a problem.

There wasn't anything I couldn't have told Mum. I knew she wouldn't overreact, that she would be practical and that she would continue to love and support me.

This made for a strong sense of security and a robust self-esteem. Mum – and Dad – conveyed to me, throughout my childhood, the belief that as long as I sincerely did my best everything would be fine.

They didn't mean I wouldn't go wrong. But honest mistakes could always – they stressed – be dealt with by a sincere apology and a determination to do better.

This advice strikes me as absolutely right. It has, anyway, stood me in good stead. One aspect of it strikes me as particular useful for a carer: I am able to forgive myself.

As every carer knows, a carer's place is in the wrong. Because we are *not* saints, we shout at our piglets, we find ourselves unable to go that extra mile and we sometimes put our own needs first. Because we are nice people this makes us feel bad. 'Here I am,' we think, 'fit and healthy (or at least not suffering from _____), and here is my poor piglet, and I couldn't even do *this* for them'.

But the only proper reply to such a thought is, 'That's right, you couldn't. It was, at that time, just a step too far.'

And what follows? That you are a wicked person? No. That you are cruel, neglectful and unworthy? No. That you couldn't, on this occasion, meet the ridiculously high standards you set yourself? Yes.

So, apologize (if necessary) and move on: everyone else would forgive you. Learning to forgive yourself is the nicest thing you can do for yourself.

> Play devil's advocate to guilt. Identify why you feel guilty ('I was so bad-tempered'/'I could have let her play with that wool'/'Why wasn't I nicer?') then challenge these beliefs: was whatever you did truly unforgiveable? Did your piglet never do something similar? Be your own best friend.

The Car

Mum was 45 when she learned to drive. Not unusual for her generation. Why should a woman drive, after all? Dad probably wasn't unusual for his generation, either. His response was to feel obsolete. That year he refused to come on holiday because he obviously wouldn't be needed.

But it was as if Mum had grown wings. She bought a rackety old Volkswagen and off she went. Her freedom wasn't complete because she had to take us with her. But we had great fun in that car.

We also learned to swear, echoing Mum with delight as, going several times around a roundabout, she swore like a trooper. She never mastered roundabouts.

Our swearing caused Mum great embarrassment. Once, visiting Dad's mother, Mum made us promise not to swear and not to eat all the cakes. But in conversation, caught between 'Isn't it a shame?' and 'Isn't it a pity?' Mum said 'Isn't it a sh***y?' then, in confusion, ate all the cakes. Richard and I had the giggles for days.

The car was Mum's escape, too. Once, uncharacteristically, she spent ages preparing a thick and probably delicious onion soup. One by one we arrived home, said we weren't hungry, and disappeared.

Mum got into her car, drove the 200 miles to her sister in Sussex and didn't come home for two weeks.

The car was instrumental in bringing home to me the fact that something was badly wrong with Mum. I went for the weekend. Mum was collecting me from the station. As I walked towards the car-park I saw Mum, looking exasperated, start the car and speed off. She must have known that I couldn't have got to her in that time. Mustn't she?

As her driving became more erratic I became more worried. I tried to persuade her to give up driving. But it was as if I were saying she should climb straight into her coffin. She wouldn't even consider it.

I was petrified she was going to kill someone (I was less worried she would kill herself – she'd have been far less distraught about that). Every time I was in the car I feared for my own life.

I proved to her that it would be cheaper for her to use a taxi whenever she went out. She ignored me. I told her she was a danger to everyone else on the road. She refused to listen. We had rows about it. I even slammed the phone down on her.

But then she crashed. She was unhurt but the car was a write-off. I shopped her to the DVLA and they took her licence away.

I recommend it if you are having the same trouble.

> Listening to other carers I hear that getting someone to give up driving is one of the hardest things we do. If you tell the DVLA about your piglet they will insist on a test. If your piglet fails ... well, that's the best argument isn't it? And it's not you making it.

Morality

An interesting (and tearing) thing about caring for someone with Alzheimer's is the constant rethinking of one's moral obligations. Is one bound to tell the truth to someone even if it will upset them and they'll have forgotten it 10 seconds later?

The 'official' view is that the person should face reality. Until I became cannier this was also my personal belief. I find it difficult to tell lies to someone I respect, and I respect my mum.

So when I found Mum in the hall, hat and coat on, telling me she was going to look for Philip, I gently explained to her that Dad had been dead for years.

Well, that wasn't much fun. Her face crumpled and she looked totally confused.

Bad enough to mourn the person you were married to for 61 years once; to do it again some years later is rotten.

I discussed the truth conundrum with Trisha, whose mum died recently. Trisha thinks the official view is nonsense. 'Why', she says, 'would I upset my mum for no reason?' Faced with her mum's desire to ring *her* long-dead mother, Trisha would pick up the phone, dial at random, listen for a bit, then tell her mum the number was engaged and they'd have to try again later. Result: happiness.

Next time Mum goes off to look for Dad I shall take her hand and suggest we go together. Then I'll take her round the block and get her talking about something else.

Another problem is whether one should keep promises made to someone who can neither remember them nor grasp the consequences of keeping them. When Mum came to live with me, she was panicky about the things I wanted to throw away. I was rash enough to promise that I would check with her before I threw anything away.

That was incredibly dumb. I don't think she had thrown away a single thing in 25 years. I swear she had every jar she'd ever opened, every plastic bag and every egg box. Then there were the knick-knacks, books and mementos. She still had my older brother's first school cap, for goodness' sake!

My practical, realistic, determined old mum would have seen immediately that everything had to go, but the new, charming, cheerful but completely out of it Mum couldn't see why anything had to: she fought me on every coffee jar. I have tried not to promise her anything since.

So do one's moral obligations lapse when a person gets Alzheimer's? Who would have guessed that caring for someone could generate such difficult philosophical problems!?

Your piglet's days of changing for the better are probably over. But you can change *yourself*. Might you learn to enjoy mess, to ignore repetition, to go with the flow? There are only two things that really matter: your piglet's safety and your sanity. Everything else is a bonus.

The Sound of Music

Mum always claimed to love opera and classical music. But she never went out of her way to listen to either. I think she felt she had to appear 'cultured'.

Nowadays she only says what she really feels. This means there's no point in listening to music unless she likes it. It is impossible to appreciate anything with Mum saying 'What a dreadful noise' or 'Can't we turn this off?' every 5 minutes.

But she does have her favourites. I've mentioned *Carmen* before. There's also the CD of Vera Lynn, George Formby and Billy Cotton. Mum loves to sing along. Then there's the Salvation Army singing popular hymns and, oddly, Ella Fitzgerald.

Actually there's not very much else Mum can do now. So, except when she's at day care, one or other of these CDs is on all the time.

This means I am now word-perfect. Even when I am not at home the blasted tunes go round and round in my head.

The other favourite is *The Sound of Music*. So when I saw that 'Sing-a-Long Sound of Music' was coming to our local theatre I booked immediately.

I expected to be bored to tears. Unexpectedly, I was enchanted. Have you ever been to one of these things? They are something of a cult. People turn up in full dress (brown paper packages tied up with string, for example, lonely goat-herds, Nazi officers and nuns) and there are prizes for the best costume. The audience ranges from 5-year-olds shyly pretending to be the youngest Von Trapp, to people even older than Mum.

The evening was led by a mistress of ceremonies. Not a job I'd envy but she did it brilliantly. We all had goodie bags and she gave us our instructions: blow the party pooper whenever a Nazi appears, for example, or say 'Aaaahhhh' every time Maria and the Count appear together ...

The point of it all was to sing along with the film. I doubt if anyone but me needed the words, but if they did there they were, appearing over the film so everyone was (literally) singing from the same song sheet.

Mum loved it. She had no idea what to do but she was happy to be jollied along by me and the people on her other side. She could neither read nor remember the words but she 'la-la-la'd with the best of them.

It may sound cringe-worthy. But it was incredibly good-natured. The trick is clearly to enter into the spirit of it. There were so many people around me doing just that I found it impossible not to.

I really enjoyed myself!

> Carers usually feel obliged to keep people informed about their piglet's condition. It can seem like yet *another* thing to do. I set up an e-mail bulletin list, so I could do the lot in one short e-mail. If you don't do e-mail, consider learning it with Whateverage (see the Resources chapter, pages 275–84).

The Perceptions of Others

You probably see it as part of your job description that your piglet's condition shouldn't ruin their life. Your piglet probably sees it as part of their job description that it shouldn't ruin yours.

But there it is. The condition. Having whatever effects it has. Inexorably. Unremittingly. Usually irreversibly. Ruining both your lives.

Ruining? Perhaps that's a step too far. Mum's Alzheimer's has changed her life. It has *not* improved it. But mostly she is relatively happy. Mum, like many with Alzheimer's, has no insight into her condition.

This isn't to say she doesn't have lucid moments, or some sort of underlying awareness. Her outbursts of frustration attest to the former, her strategies for hiding her confusion and memory loss, the latter. But Mum usually succeeds, as she always has done, in finding things to be happy about.

Other carers are not so lucky. Some people have a talent for misery. Sometimes these people get Alzheimer's too. Caring for them must be unbelievably grim. I couldn't do it. With Mum at least I am not the only person trying to see the bright side.

Mum's Alzheimer's isn't ruining my life, either. Certainly there are things I'd rather be doing than coping with it. But given that the Alzheimer's exists, and there's nothing we can do about it, I am actively choosing to help Mum deal with it. She could, after all, go into a home.

At lunch the other day I was sitting next to someone who, learning about Mum, assumed I was depressed. I found this irritating. Even more irritating was this woman's attempt to cheer me up. I felt like pinning her to the ground and shouting '*I do not need cheering up.*'

Why is it that in such situations it always sounds as if one is protesting too much?

Later, rather shaken by the strength of my response, I reflected on whether I *wasn't* protesting too much. Am I depressed? I don't think so. I really don't think so. I am not usually unaware of my own moods and emotions. On the contrary, I think I am quite good at recognizing and responding to my own needs.

I think my irritation was prompted by the fact that this woman had no experience of Alzheimer's, of caring, or of *me*. Her belief I was depressed was based simply on the belief that anyone caring for someone with Alzheimer's must be depressed.

But this assumes that she can lump into one category everyone caring for someone with Alzheimer's. As if their situations are identical. As if their uniqueness as people is irrelevant. As if, somehow, they have stopped *being* people.

Wouldn't *you* have been irritated?

I prefer to think of myself as having chosen to care for Mum. It gives me control, makes me feel less of a victim. I could have put her in a home. You could do the same. Instead we are voluntarily doing what we believe to be right. Nice!

Dignity

Last week we had builders in. I asked them to come at 9.30 so Mum would be out before they arrived. But at 8.15, pleading light traffic, they were here. Mum was in the bath, the cats hadn't been fed, and I was in my dressing gown.

By 9.30 Mum had several times fallen over their tools, charmingly asked them who they were 50 times, panicked at every loud noise and asked what was going on every other second. They were squirming with guilt and I was enjoying that 'I told you so' feeling.

When we'd talked times, the man in charge had made soothing noises about understanding my situation. It made me think he must be a carer. He turned out to have young children.

People often assume that caring for Mum must be like caring for a child. I can see there are similarities. But the differences are profound enough to make the comparison misleading (and irritating).

With children there are the compensations: the heart-melting hug, the wonderful scent of their scalps, the flashes of promise, the constant acquisition of new skills …

With Mum it mostly works the other way. There is the odd heart-melting hug, but flashes of lucidity are not comparable to flashes of promise, she's constantly losing rather than gaining skills, and as for scent: well, let's not go there!

Children, furthermore, are a life project. In caring for them one is fulfilling part of one's own life-plan. But my life-plan certainly didn't include caring for Mum. I care for her because she needs it, not because that's the way I want it.

Then there's the fact that children and their needs are largely catered for. You may think facilities for children are poor, but from where I am sitting they look fantastic. I should love to send Mum to school every day, or put her in a crèche. Changing facilities, dedicated entertainment, menus and activities would make my life – and Mum's – so much easier.

The big thing, though, is dignity. Children accept you care for them, that their lives are largely directed by you and that you make decisions for them. To a child this represents security (even if it is irksome).

But Mum has no insight into her condition. She believes she is totally competent. This means that she does not accept I care for her. She thinks she cares for me, or that we simply share a house. When I direct Mum's activities, or make decisions for her, the world – to her – has gone topsy-turvy. In a most distressing way. I see no direct equivalent to this in caring for a child.

Yes, children gibe against authority. But they are struggling for the joy of control, not desperately fending off the loss of it. Their control grows. Mum's diminishes.

It is one of the most difficult things I have to negotiate.

It might help in darker times to spend an hour going through your piglet's day from your piglet's perspective. What must it feel like to wake up and not know where you are? To spend your days with those you perceive to be strangers? To never know what you are doing or why? To find complete strangers making all your decisions for you?

Deterioration

Mum had her MOT last week. Usually they invite me along. This year when they rang, my younger brother was here. He said he didn't want to go and then failed to tell me they'd rung. (Can anyone explain brothers?)

The first I heard about it was when they rang with the results. Apparently Mum didn't deteriorate at all last year. Indeed, if anything, she got better.

Well! All that shows is how useless the tests are. They are totally dependent on how the person is on the day. On some days Mum can't remember her own name. On other days she'll irritatingly remember something I'd rather she didn't.

Last year Mum couldn't spell for toffee, apparently. This year she was able to spell the word they gave her. She was also – wait for it – *able to spell it backwards!* Could you do that? No, nor could I.

The physical tests are also useless, underestimating the desire to please. If I asked Mum to jump in the air she'd tell me I was daft. Let someone in a white coat ask her and she'll do it twice to show willing.

So do *I* think she has deteriorated in the past year? You bet I do. She's now losing skills that were key to her ability to engage in meaningful interaction.

Until relatively recently, for example, she was able to answer 'small talk' gambits immediately, appropriately and convincingly. This meant others warmed to her before, inevitably, discovering her limitations.

Now she is losing her grip on pronouns. So if someone asks her, 'How are you?' she won't be sure whom they're talking to. I think she thinks that 'you' means the other person (i.e. not her, if you see what I mean).

She can no longer follow simple instructions, either. Yesterday, for example, she wanted to turn on the lamp. This particular lamp has a switch on its base. 'Move your hand to the base of the lamp,' I said, 'No, the *base*, the *bottom*, the bit on the *floor*.' Mum started to look flustered, then accidentally put her hand on the switch.

'That's right,' I said quickly, 'Now press the switch.' 'What?' said Mum, and moved her hand away. I gave up and did it for her.

When, drying up, she wants to know where things go, I used to be able to say 'in the cupboard' or 'behind the microwave'. Now she has no idea what I mean and has to guess. She gets it wrong ten times before getting it right. So having her help me has become hugely labour-intensive. But she loves to help. And it gives her something to do. So I grit my teeth and carry on.

I think I should get a medal.

When Mum first moved in I had a list of jobs for her. She ironed, dried the dishes, helped make beds and hang out washing, drew curtains and plumped up cushions. But I wish I'd been more aware as she lost these skills. I am sure I would have been able to replace them with others, rather than leaving her feeling useless.

Dad

Mum and Dad had, in effect, two families. Christopher and Judy in 1940 and 1944 respectively, then me in 1955 and Richard in 1957. Two boy/girl pairs. But here the resemblance ends.

Christopher and Judy were war babies, brought up by Mum whilst Dad was fighting. Mum (20 when she had Christopher) and Dad (23 when he was called up) were still growing up themselves.

When Dad came home in 1946 he was, according to Mum, 'impossible'. Wanting to establish himself as *pater familias* he tried to impose his authority.

He once decided, for example, that he needed Christopher's ration egg more than Christopher did. So he took it. Mum, standing behind him, said it was the final straw. She hit him smartly on the head with a spoon.

The BOINGGG!!! it made, and Dad's bellow of pain, followed her as she rushed to the loo and locked herself in. She refused to come out until he agreed to drop the Acting Major Talbot bit.

Similar scenarios must have been playing out all over the land.

By the mid-1950s, family life largely established, Mum decided she wanted another baby. Two, indeed, because one would get desperately spoiled. Against Dad's better judgement, I was soon on the way.

Dad took to being a proper father like a duck to water. Because Mum was busy getting qualifications, in fact, Richard and I were largely brought up by him.

He took his duties seriously. On Saturdays, as he made his own breakfast, he would make us our 'strips': half slices of fried bread lovingly spread with egg yolk and bits of bacon, sausage, egg white and tomato. Then we had 'specials' – small bowls of jelly babies, dolly mixtures and Maltesers. These were the only sweets Dad allowed. Mum's rules were different – a fact we exploited mercilessly.

Then we would sit beside him on the sofa while he read our comics: *The Robin* for me, *The Eagle* for Richard. Dad was brilliant at the voices and the noises (whizz! whoosh! KERRpoinggg!).

Next he would mark the 'homework' he had set us. Each of us had a notebook in which Dad would painstakingly have written out a number of questions: '244 – 37 = ?', 'The hero of *Moby Dick* = ?', 'The famous river in Egypt = ?', 'Write a short essay on …'. His satisfaction when we got it right was palpable.

I still have these books, complete with Dad's comments. When I come across them it is almost as if he is beside me. But when Dad suddenly developed dementia after a stroke, I didn't even consider caring for him in the way I care for Mum.

I still get pangs of guilt.

If your piglet can't go on public transport unaccompanied, you might be able to get a card entitling you to free public transport when you accompany them. You will need to get a doctor's letter to confirm they need to be accompanied. Contact your Council.

Coeliac Disease

I don't think I have mentioned before that Mum has coeliac disease? This means that she can't eat gluten – no wheat, rye or barley. To put it more meaningfully: bread, pastry, cakes, batter, biscuits and cereal are all off-limits.

I can't tell you how much of a pain this is.

If we go out, for example, I have to take supplies. You can bet your boots that otherwise she won't be able to eat anything. Buffets, for example, are a real ordeal – sausage rolls, sandwiches, pizza slices, breaded ham, pastries, cake ... Poor Mum: eating is one of the few pleasures she has left.

So that Mum can occasionally enjoy some of these things, I bake. Yes, bake. In my spare time.

Mum was fine until she was 70. Annoyingly, this means that her new diet didn't have time to 'take' before the Alzheimer's set in. So Mum doesn't remember that she can't eat these staple (and much-loved) foods. I have to watch her like a hawk.

I am forever whipping biscuits out of her very mouth, for example, just as she has said to the person offering it, 'Oh, how kind, I'd love one.' You can imagine the looks I get.

And the comments: 'Oh, can't she just have one?' they'll say. 'Yes,' says Mum, 'surely one can't hurt?'

But one *will* hurt. Coeliac disease is not a food intolerance, it is a condition in which the intestine cannot process gluten. When Mum eats it she gets a painful rash, which is horrible for her. She also gets diarrhoea, which is horrible for me.

I feel like a bully when I refuse her 'just one'. There's no point in saying, 'You'll thank me' because of course she won't; she just thinks I am being mean. So does everyone else.

Restaurants don't help. This weekend, Mum went for a pub lunch with her brothers. They were assured by the chef that there was no gluten in rye bread.

WRONG!

So I'm in for a bad week.

I should, of course, as a service to other coeliacs, write to the pub. I should also write to the restaurant who assured me last week that pasta is gluten-free. Then there are all those helpful people who think spelt is wheat-free. But if I were to write to everyone who gets it wrong, I'd do nothing else.

The fashion for food intolerances has made my life easier in some ways. There is far more gluten-free food available for example. In other ways it has made it more difficult because people have become sceptical.

I would like to hang a notice around Mum's neck. I wonder if people would think me less of a bully?

> You probably know this already, but just in case ... never go out with your piglet without your emergency kit: spare disposable pants, change of clothes, something to eat and drink (special diets catered for), in winter one of those things that warm up when you open the pack and in summer a tiny personal fan.

Care Costs

It looks as if I am going to get Direct Payments!

This means that the County Council will allocate a sum of money to me to cover some of the costs of Mum's care. What a relief this will be.

Given that Mum can't be left alone, I can only go out if she is at Willows, her day care centre, or if someone comes in to look after her. Willows is only open between 10 a.m. and 3 p.m., so I turn into a pumpkin at about 2.30 to get home in time for the bus. It doesn't make for a great social life (makes work difficult, too).

But I am determined to have a social life. This is for Mum's sake as much as mine. I dread to think what I'd be like with her if I didn't get out occasionally.

I have a good system for getting friends and family to help (see my Tips for Carers, starting on page 219) but mostly I have to use them for work. For my social life, therefore, I use professional carers. But they cost a minimum of £10–£15 per hour.

Going for a pizza with friends, therefore, costs me £25 for the meal and £60 for the carer (7 p.m. until 10 p.m. for the evening, plus half an hour's travelling time each way). Eighty-five quid for a 'cheap' night out! Not many nights in a month I can do this.

Then sometimes I have to work at weekends, and can't get friends or relatives to help. For the privilege of working over the weekend it costs me a minimum of £120, but more likely £180.

My weekend's pay is £81.

I don't pay all care costs myself. Mum contributes £70 per week. She can't afford more because she is on the minimum income guarantee. But it helps.

But isn't it the pits? You wouldn't believe that carers save the government £87 billion a year – *£87 billion! Every year!*

I think I'll organize a carers' strike. We would take our piglets to the nearest hospital (shopping centre, train station – all suggestions welcome) and simply leave them. We'd inform the media so there'd be heart-rending pictures of abandoned piglets in every newspaper and on every television channel. On every radio station piglets would be being interviewed (that'd be fun).

But what should we demand to end our strike? It would be marvellous just to get what we're entitled to. But perhaps we should be more ambitious? Perhaps we should ask for some reasonable percentage of what we're really worth?

The real risk is that, having relieved ourselves of our caring responsibilities, we wouldn't want to go back.

Dear oh dear ... what would the State do then?

> If your piglet has a severe mental impairment and gets one of a quite long list of benefits (like attendance allowance) they will not be included for Council Tax purposes. This means that if it's just you and your piglet you get a 25 per cent discount because you 'live alone'. Contact your local Council for more info.

Caring for Other People's Money

Throughout our childhood Dad managed to give Mum, me and my siblings the impression that the wolf's nose was on the threshold. We didn't even bother to ask for anything we didn't need. As he got older, his worry increased. The maintenance of the house particularly exercised him. He kept it in tip-top condition. But as he became older he felt it was running away with him and that the roof would fall in any moment.

So when he had his stroke I assumed that if there was any money at all, it was enough only for the basics.

As Dad didn't have an Enduring Power of Attorney [more on this later in the Practicalities chapters], this was my impression for the three months it took the Court of Protection to award me the Receivership. Until then, not being able to access his accounts, I had no idea how things actually stood.

In the meantime Dad had gone into a nursing home, the fees for which were £650 per week. I was beside myself with dread. How on Earth were my parents to live?

When I learned about how charges for nursing homes worked, I was able to relax a bit.

The idea that people have to sell their homes to pay a spouse's nursing home fees is largely a myth to which the less responsible parts of the media subscribe when in shock-horror mode. I read it often and it infuriates me. It was, and is, completely false. So long as Mum was living in the house there was no chance it would have to be sold. What a relief!

Then, on getting the Receivership, I learned my parents were comfortable enough financially so long as the roof didn't actually fall in. They owned their small house and they had a modest, painfully accumulated portfolio of savings and investments.

But, as I imagine is the case with most people, it was not possible to pay a professional to look after their money. So I had to learn to muddle through.

Until this point my financial dealings had consisted largely of discussing my overdraft with my bank. I spent sleepless nights worrying myself sick about the responsibility. My days were full of anxious discussions with building societies, banks and utility companies. I didn't even know which questions to ask, never mind which decisions to make. I had no idea how to evaluate the information I was given.

Some of the decisions I made: Oh, boy!

For example, Dad held a small number of shares in a company that had once been owned by the only Talbot ever to make money. I sold them at the very bottom of the market. Why? Because I was frightened of them.

How sensible is that?

> If your piglet has been diagnosed fairly recently do not assume that they cannot any longer sign an Enduring Power of Attorney or a third-party mandate, or appoint a permanent agent (to access a post office account). Check with your solicitor before approaching the dreaded Court of Protection. See pages 235–48 for more on this.

Euston Station

As a carer you quickly learn that your life is not your own. Neither is your house. Or your time. Everyone else, it seems, enjoys their 'me' time, but you go through life as if it were a three-legged race.

Before Mum came to live with me I revelled in my independence. Most of my life I have lived alone and loved it. Life was busy and exciting, but whenever I needed to I could close my front door and be blissfully solitary.

Now my house is like Euston Station. There's always someone here or about to arrive. There's Mum's hairdresser, chiropodist, psychiatric social worker and care manager. Then there are all the people who come to see her: siblings, grandchildren, old friends and general well-wishers. All need to be greeted, offered refreshments, made comfortable and chaperoned.

The chaperoning is a recent thing. Despite the Alzheimer's Mum's always been good at the social stuff. For ages I've been aware that she has no idea who most of these people are, but she's generally managed to hide this by being so delighted to see them (whoever they are). She's very life-enhancing, my mum.

But she's losing her grip. She's not been able, for a long time, to answer simple questions ('Do you still go to church?', 'Where did you live before?'). Until recently, however, people didn't notice because, when questioned, Mum would start paying extravagant compliments ('What a lovely dress!', 'How nicely you smile!'). People found it a bit disconcerting, but hey!

Now, as her mind fragments further, she can't do this. She knows there's something she's not doing, and this makes her defensive. For the first time ever her sunniness is being overshadowed by defensiveness. In company now she'll often retreat into a shell and say nothing. Not every visitor can cope. Hence the chaperoning (though I sometimes fear that by filling the gap I'm making it worse).

Poor Mum. She has always seen it as a duty – albeit a pleasant one – to keep the conversational ball rolling. I think she feels she's letting herself down. Sometimes she looks really miserable.

She is also more frightened generally than she used to be. This is making her uncharacteristically clingy. I have taken to bathing when she's at day care because otherwise, as soon as I'm in the bath, Mum's upstairs asking where I am. In fact, whenever I go out of the room nowadays Mum'll be at my heels in minutes wanting to know where I am.

It is very wearing. It's clear, in fact, that I am soon going to need a lot more help with Mum.

Do you think I'll get it? I'll keep you informed ...

Is your piglet suddenly clinging? Do not give in. Go out without hesitating. Then put them out of your mind. Better this than to spin it out creating more misery all round. To let this behaviour get a grip is to set yourself up for a life of misery. Warning: this is (much) easier said than done.

Respite

I hear on the radio that The Alzheimer's Society is warning that care homes don't know how to deal with people with dementia.

Too right they don't.

A year ago the Council gave me six weeks a year respite. Mum would go into a home for a week at a time and I could do what I liked.

Bliss! I had a wonderful time the first week. But then Mum came home.

I went to greet her as the bus arrived and saw her face, white and drawn, staring out of the window. She saw me, put both hands out as if reaching for me, and burst into tears.

For four hours she cried, saying repeatedly she hated herself, was a bad person, and wanted to die.

What had they done to my mum?

Not only was she traumatized, she was filthy. She had impacted faeces in her fingernails, and can't have been changed for days. Her bra was missing, as were her teeth. Later I discovered she had a urine infection. She also had the painful rash that comes from eating gluten. Half her clothes were missing, as was a precious family photograph.

For five weeks I comforted her, telling her she wasn't a bad person and that everyone loved her. So did the day care people (who were horrified by her state). At night I had to look under the bed and in the wardrobe before I could leave her, and she was petrified of having baths.

One respite week. Five weeks serious hands-on care and a lot of misery. Bad deal.

I complained, of course. But it was pointless. An 'independent' investigator (from head office) was sent in. She assured me she was doing everything, and promised to discuss her final report with me.

I never saw her again. Months later I received the report. It said Mum must have had the urine infection before she arrived, and the rash was a mystery because she hadn't eaten gluten. She had herself chosen not to wear her bra and teeth, and she had been clean when she left the home and must have become dirty on the journey. Her upset, they said, was because she was used to getting one-to-one care from me.

They assured me, however, their systems for logging possessions were being reviewed.

I could have taken my complaint to the next stage. I wrote saying I was unhappy. They replied this was 'unhelpful'. Shamefully, I gave up. I was hugely stressed and just couldn't face it. How are carers supposed to deal with this *as well?*

So I think The Alzheimer's Society should go for it – all power to them. I cancelled the rest of my respite care, and have since heard of many other carers doing the same.

Our first respite might not have been so disastrous if we'd started when we should have done: two years earlier.
But I didn't discover we were entitled before then. If we'd started when we could have, Mum wouldn't have been as vulnerable. I would have been less in need of a total break. Are you entitled? As I write this, the Government has announced a sum of £400 million to be put aside for respite care. Contact Social Services. But plan properly. See pages 267–68 for more.

Charing Cross

Last Thursday night I woke in a panic. I had committed myself to something crazy: the following day I was to take Mum, by train, to Kent to stay with her brother and sister-in-law.

I must have been mad to suggest this. What's more – and incredibly I hadn't realized this until now – we were travelling through London on a Friday *at rush hour!*

This had been in my diary for ages, but I had been too busy to take on board the full implications. At 2 a.m. the full implications were staring me in the face. They kept me awake for two hours.

In the morning, without high expectations, I rang London station assistance … and got through straight away. I told the charming young woman who answered that I needed to book a wheelchair for my elderly mum. She took my details and said she'd ring as soon as she had booked it.

Again – such cynicism – my expectations were low. But 5 minutes later there she was promising there'd be a wheelchair waiting at the entrance to Charing Cross station at 4.10 p.m.

So now I only had to get to Charing Cross.

At 3 a.m. I had decided that all I could do was throw money at the problem. Instead of walking to the bus that would take us to Victoria (Mum: 'How long must I do this? Can I sit down? I'm exhausted') we took a taxi. As we arrived at the bus stop, so did the bus!

On the bus I read Mum's cat-watching book to her, and told her 100 times we were going to stay with Ian and Betty. The nearer we got to London the more nervous I became.

But we succeeded immediately in getting a taxi, went straight to Charing Cross, and arrived an hour before we needed to. So we went into the big hotel on the station.

Two glasses of wine later (one was for Mum, but having asked for it she didn't want it – honest) at 4.10 exactly we appeared at the entrance to Charing Cross … and there was the wheelchair!

The man pushing it – Alan Baldwin – couldn't have been nicer. He took us to buy tickets (we went straight to the front of the queue), then to the right platform, then he helped us onto the train. Without him it would have been a nightmare negotiating the commuters intent on getting away for the weekend. As it was I was able to relax, slightly sozzled, and answer Mum's question ('Where are we going?') another 100 times before we arrived at our station to be collected by Ian (who also gave us a lift home).

I still can't believe it!

Have you noticed, when out and about, that your piglet is reluctant to climb stairs with those black and yellow 'warnings' strips? Having thought about it I suspect they see only the black and yellow, interpreting the rest of the step as a hole. How would you feel about climbing stairs only 2 inches wide?

Bedtime

Until I was 11 Mum used to put me and my brother Richard to bed at 6.30 p.m. Even in mid-summer. I used to lie in bed, the sun streaming in, listening to the other children play. Cruelty, I call it.

When quizzed about it later she said, without a hint of shame, that by 6.30 she couldn't bear another minute of us.

Another trick she had was whisking us to bed during an advertisement break. That stopped once I learned to read 'End of Part One'. I have a vivid memory of her groaning that she wished I'd never learned to read.

But what goes around comes around. Now I can't wait to get her to bed. As it gets dark by 4 at the moment, I can often have her done and dusted by 7.30. It's brilliant.

Of course where, on me, she just asserted her adult rights, I have to be more subtle.

So at about 5.30 I start yawning and saying I wouldn't mind an early night. In her companionable way, she'll say 'What a good idea!' or 'That sounds good to me.' If I'm lucky she'll even start yawning.

Then after supper, we watch the news. I say several times 'Shall we go to bed when the news has finished?' Mum has no concept of time but 'bed after the news' makes sense: she and Dad always watched *News at Ten* before going to bed. Again, despite her night-owl tendencies, she'll make some positive response.

But often I don't even wait until the news has finished. I have a nifty little gadget that stops live television, allowing you to play it later. At the first advertisement break, therefore, I hit the button, and say 'Bedtime! Will you help me wash up first?' She's so pleased to help that she doesn't even think of protesting. Then she goes up like a lamb.

But if she was mean to do it to me (and she was), am I being mean to do it to her?

I'm afraid I don't care. It's such a relief to get her to bed and have a bit of time to myself that I am beyond the moral niceties. It means I can read the paper without being interrupted every five seconds (by the same question), or watch television without Mum's blankly uncomprehending commentary. Or I can catch up with some work without having to check on her every minute, or ring a friend without feeling guilty that Mum's feeling left out.

What worries me is that I won't be able to do this in summer when the sun is streaming in through the window.

I think I'll have to buy some black-out blinds.

> Isn't it so irritating sometimes that everything revolves around your piglet? They *always* come first. 'What about me?' you yearn to say. Don't push this question away. Your piglet *shouldn't* always come first. There are times when *you* matter more: after all, what would your piglet do without you?

Through Her Eyes

Imagine waking up tomorrow ... in a strange room, one you've never been in before. You've no idea why you're here or how you got here.

You pretend you're still asleep, keeping an ear open for a hint. No hint is forthcoming. But you start realizing that some things are familiar ... those photographs, for example, don't you know those people?

If you do, you don't know their names. Or who they are.

But you feel you ought to know who they are.

That makes you feel stupid. In fact, as you lie there, you feel more stupid by the minute – how can your mind be so blank?

Eventually you feel you must get up. Someone must know why you're here.

There are some clothes on the chair. But what if they're not yours? Better go down as you are.

You set off downstairs, politely calling 'Hello?' as you go. To your relief a woman bowls out, greeting you as if you're expected. She acts as if she knows you. This is odd because you're not sure you know her.

Before you know it, though, she's whisked you upstairs, undressed you, washed and dressed you. It's all very confusing. Then you're back downstairs being made to take some pills. There's an awful lot of them and you've no idea what they're for. Can this be right?

The woman doesn't take your protests seriously, and she seems to be in a hurry. She keeps telling you the bus is about to arrive as if you know what that means. Are you supposed to be going somewhere? If so, where? Why? And with whom?

When will you be allowed home? Where is home, actually? Try as you might you can't remember where you belong. The only thing you know is that it isn't here.

The woman is getting more stressed by the minute; she's dashing in and out, making you feel quite jumpy. The bus is late, apparently. You wish it would come because her stress is making you stressed. Is it your fault the bus is late?

Finally it comes. Before you know it you've been bundled into a coat, had a hat crammed on your head, and you're being frog-marched towards a bus full of old people. For the next hour you're driven all over the place collecting even more old people.

Still no one tells you what this is all about.

Imagine that this goes on all day every day. Whenever you ask whether you shouldn't be going home, people laugh and tell you you're already home. You never feel certain you

*know what's going on, and everyone else seems to be living
life around you.* I'd go nuts. Wouldn't you? Tell me: how
does Mum remain so cheerful?

> Find an hour. Pour a glass of wine. List everything your
> piglet does that drives you bonkers. Try viewing each in
> a different light. Is it time-wasting? No, it's time spent
> making your piglet feel better. Is it messy? No, it's glorious
> abandon! Aim to swap angst for a glow of virtue!

Christmas

It's Christmas Eve. The tree is decorated and sparkling with
lights. The (gluten-free) cake is marzipanned and iced. It's even
decorated: the icing Christmas tree is a bit wonky and I wish I
knew how to get icing smooth, but it looks OK (tastes OK, too –
I've been feeding it brandy for a month!).

We have carols playing and Mum is la-la-ing to them, the cat
purring fatly beside her. When I tell her it's Christmas Eve, she
exclaims with delight.

Sound idyllic? In fact it's all smoke and mirrors.

I haven't sent any Christmas cards. Couldn't face the
envelopes. For three years I've intended to type everything into
my computer so I can just print off labels. But despite being on
my 'to do' list for yet another year, it's still not done.

My cousin boasts he only sends cards every three years. He
reckons that's enough not to get scrubbed off everyone's list. I
hope he's right.

As for tomorrow: I am sharing Christmas with friends, and I
have baggsied the easy bit.

Tomorrow, 11 people will come to mine at 1 p.m. for champagne, smoked salmon, olives, melon and prosciutto. The
champagne is chilling, the smoked salmon pre-sliced, the bread

sliced by the baker, the olives bought from the expensive local deli and the melon and prosciutto will be dead easy.

We'll open presents, accompanied by more carols. Then, leaving the washing up for later, we'll go in convoy to Felicity and Ian's house a mile away.

It'll be a full traditional Christmas: roast turkey with all the trimmings, followed by (gluten-free) Christmas pud and brandy butter. Then when we're feeling peckish a couple of hours later we'll have cake, mince pies, chocolate, fruit, etc., before turkey sandwiches for supper. Pretty much what you're having I expect.

As well as the cake, I am providing sprouts, parsnips and (gluten-free) bread sauce. Richard and Trish, from South Africa, are bringing wine and champagne. Felicity's sister Liz from Canada has been here for a few days and she and Felicity have done the lion's share of the work. As well as Mum and Felicity's dad, Gordon, there'll be three teenage boys, Oliver, Rob and James, on whose appetites we're relying.

Mum will be in seventh heaven. She adores Ian, who always greets her with a huge hug and talks to her as if she is a real person, as does Felicity. She'll also get to flirt with Gordon, who is wonderful with her. There'll even be four two-month-old puppies to get under everyone's feet.

I'll do what ought, in my book, to be done at Christmas time – go to church (before Mum gets up), eat too much, drink too much, and relax with the people I love.

May your Christmas be as good!

If your piglet is like Mum, traditional times like Christmas are a real boon. Thrust a cracker at Mum and she knows exactly what to do. Give her a gaily wrapped present and she'll immediately open it. Say 'Happy Christmas!' and she'll say it right back. How wonderful for her to know what she is doing.

A Disgraced Fatcat

Fatcat is in disgrace.

It has been cold here. Fatcat doesn't like the cold. In particular she can't see any reason, when it is cold, to go outside. She'd rather pee in comfort. So she does.

She always goes either under the desk in my study or in the corner of Mum's bedroom.

I then have to arm myself with a basin full of water, two rags, a scrubbing brush, the stain remover and two old pillowcases. Then I blot as much as I can – horrible job – spray the rest, then scrub. Finally I spray again and cover the stain with the pillowcases and something heavy for 12 hours or so.

What a palaver!

Every time I have to do it I get EXTREMELY irritated. Sometimes I can't stop myself taking it out on Mum.

'That b***dy cat of yours,' I say, 'it's peed on the carpet again.' 'Oh,' says Mum, looking horrified, 'she's never done that before.' 'Oh yes, she has,' I spit, 'she does it all the time and I'm sick of it.'

But then Mum gets really distressed. I can see that she is worried I might do something to the cat.

Put a bung in it, perhaps?

Jolly good idea. But no. The cat leads a charmed life. So long as Mum is around she will be fed, brushed and watered. By me, of course. The only thing I can't bear is cleaning up after her.

No, that's not true. I also get fed up with finding bits of stuff everywhere. I have just scraped up half a squashed macaroon from the sitting-room carpet. Macaroon must be one of the few things Fatcat won't eat.

It's not that Mum thinks I starve her (I don't think). It's more that Mum can't resist Fatcat's begging. She has such a low centre of gravity that she can sit on her haunches, waving her paws and looking appealing. I think it's gross. But Mum just melts.

Poor old Fatcat is the same age as Oedipus. But Oedipus can leap elegantly onto the back of the sofa without apparent effort. The best Fatcat can do is put her front paws on the sofa, heave herself up bit by bit until her back legs are on, then pantingly flop. Soon she'll be asleep, her huge tum protruding, snoring heavily.

When Fatcat first arrived I took her to the vet. He looked disapproving and said she must lose 4 kg. I put her on a diet. This did not make me popular. After two years Fatcat had lost – ooh, 2 oz?

I gave up (and haven't taken her to the vet since). Would anyone like a (very) large tabby?

> Funeral plans: Dad took out one for himself and one for Mum after he had his first stroke. They cost £9 a month each. Dad lived for another 15 years, Mum for 23 years. That's a total of over £1,600 paid in for Dad's, and nearly £2,500 for Mum's. Each plan paid out about £700. If I had let them lapse we wouldn't have got even this. If only they'd put their £18 a month into a savings account.

Christmas Presents

It's unbelievable. It's Monday, the day Mum doesn't go to day care. Usually I continually have to find Mum something to do. She'll take up whatever I suggest for 2 minutes, then discard it and look around for something else.

I have learned to prepare for Mondays (and Sundays, when there is also no day care). I save up the ironing, for example. If Mum does three items at a time I can ask her if she'll help me iron about ten times throughout the day. That's helpful.

Then there's the drying up: it's amazing how much two adults and two cats can generate if you try hard enough. Then there's the feeding of the cats. But that only happens twice a day and takes 2 minutes, however much I spin it out.

Try as I might there are many times in the day when Mum looks bored to death.

But not today. Today she is engrossed in a book. Absolutely glued to it. Every few minutes she laughs with delight. She keeps telling me I must read it, it's the best thing she's ever read and it is really important.

I am looking at her now. She is completely silent (bliss!), eating the book with her eyes, a lovely smile playing on her face.

The book? It's called *Ethel and Ernest* by Raymond Briggs – he of *The Snowman* fame. It was given to Mum for Christmas by Judy, my sister. An inspired present!

It is incredibly touching. It tells, in cartoons, the story of Briggs' parents: how they met, married, weathered the war, brought up their son, then eventually died.

We enjoy their courtship and their pride in their first house, delight with them when their son arrives, share their family jokes, and recognize (or at least I do) his dad's socialist tendencies and his mum's snobbishness. We sympathize with their sense that the world is running away from them, and feel their son's grief when they die.

It is very much the story of Mum's life with Dad: the very ordinariness of it speaks to most of us with an echo of our own childhood.

Judy was obviously on a roll buying presents this year. She also bought Mum a calendar with a tiger on each page: tigers playing in snow, tigers stalking through undergrowth, tigers swimming in rivers and so on.

Mum adores tigers (it started with an inspired present of my own: an adopted tiger), and this calendar hit the spot exactly. It kept her happy all Christmas day. It is now in the upstairs loo. I hear Mum exclaim every time she goes in.

I am ashamed to say I recycled the scarf I gave Mum last year.

> Save yourself time and energy. When you are in the mood for cooking, and can do it (perhaps with your piglet's 'help'), double, triple or quadruple quantities and freeze the excess in piglet portions or you-and-piglet portions. Then when you don't feel like cooking, grab a frozen portion, microwave it and Bob's your uncle!

Transport

I don't know what has happened to the 'special transport service' around here. It used to be fantastic. But that was probably because of the regular driver, Ray, who was a complete star: always happy to help and always prepared to be flexible.

If I was going to be late, for example, I could ring and ask him if he would leave Mum until last. If he could he'd happily do so.

But Ray, sadly for the carers around here, was promoted. (Well deserved – congratulations, Ray.) Since then the system seems to have collapsed.

Before, for example, I could be reasonably sure that the bus would arrive between 9.30 and 10. This meant that I would start getting Mum up at 8.45ish and, once she'd washed, dressed and had breakfast, she wouldn't have long to wait for the bus. She'd go off to Willows and I would go off to work. This ate into my day, but it didn't stress me out because it was reasonably predictable.

Then we were warned that the bus might arrive earlier or later than usual. This sounded worrying, but now I am actually dealing with it I think of it as the most stressful thing I have to deal with as a carer.

The bus occasionally arrives as early as 8.45. This means Mum has to start getting up at 8 a.m. just in case. But then sometimes the bus doesn't arrive until *10.30*. So Mum, having finished her breakfast for 8.45, is sitting there twiddling her thumbs for an hour and a quarter.

It means that even though sometimes the bus comes early, I can't rely on it. So I can't arrange meetings or any serious work for the morning because I might end up letting everyone down. It also means I might have to amuse Mum for over an hour. This is not only extremely difficult, it also prevents me doing anything useful in the house. My mornings are now largely a waste of time.

My afternoons are also largely a waste of time, thanks to the new system. Although I must be at home by 3.30 in case Mum gets back, she sometimes doesn't get back until 4.30 or even 5. A whole chunk of my afternoon is spent doing virtually nothing.

DOESN'T ANYONE REALIZE HOW BUSY I AM?

I am not the only local carer who feels like this. We feel that whoever is now organizing the system is treating us with contempt. Anyone who attached any value to us and our needs would not arrange the system like this.

I thought that writing this might be therapeutic. Actually it's made me hopping mad!

If only I had been able to drive at this point. Predictability is so incredibly important to a carer. Especially a working carer. Our lives are planned to the last minute: there is no room for unpredictability. Some professional carers realize this and make a point of being on time. Others don't.

Mismanagement

Oh, goodness gracious me – I am tearing my hair out here. I have mismanaged things, and poor old Mum is taking the flak.

Three weeks ago I finally heard I'd be getting Direct Payments backdated to 2nd November. On 11th January, therefore, a lump sum of over £5,000 landed in the special account I'd set up. The Council will add to this at the rate of – wait for it – £403 per week.

£403 per week! Whoopee!

This will completely revolutionize my life. It will enable me to *have* a life. It is completely wonderful.

But the freedom went straight to my head. I immediately arranged with an agency for carers to come Tuesdays to Fridays from 8.15 to whenever the bus for day care comes (which could be any time at all), and from 3.30 when it (might) come back until 5.30 when I'll get back.

My plan was that, free from the stress of waiting for the bus, I could leave the house at 8.30 and return at 5.30. Maybe I could even get some work done.

For two weeks I did just that. I set myself up with my laptop in a corner of the café in a local bookshop. At lunchtime I took a short walk, read the paper, then went back to the bookshop. Then I'd go for a swim. Complete bliss.

In the meantime, though, unbeknownst to me, Mum's life was unravelling.

I was dimly aware there were a huge number of carers, rather than the 'small team' I had been promised. I certainly noticed they were nearly always late. Then there was the one who took Mum's paper to read herself!

Then the wonderful people at Willows rang to say Mum seemed depressed and needed changing a lot. They suggested she might have a urine infection. 'Aargh!' I thought, 'I don't have time to take her to the doctor.'

The penny didn't drop even when, getting home 5 minutes late, I found Mum on her own. The carer had simply gone.

From all this I averted my eyes, so desperate was I to keep my work schedule intact.

But things have become unignorable. Mum is completely distraught. She even says she wants to kill herself. I can finally see that for the last three weeks I have been treating her as a *thing*, an object to be moved around at *my* direction, to enable *me* to work. I feel dreadful.

I have cancelled everything for both of us this week. I shall devote the week to getting us back to square one. Then I'll make a proper Mum-orientated plan.

It must be possible, with all this money, for Mum to get the care she deserves at the same time as my being able to work.

> Looking back I see that this was the beginning of the end. I was given the Direct Payments in recognition of the fact that something had to be done. But actually something should have been done at least three months earlier. I believe it was the administration attached to the Direct Payments that finished me off.

Agony

What a terrible week. The debacle with care over the last three weeks has come home to roost.

Mum can't bear me being out of her sight. If I leave the room she's on my heels in seconds, calling 'Is anyone here?' It makes me want to weep. She wants constant attention, too. If I try to do something – read the paper, do a bit of work – within 5 minutes she's looking like a wet weekend, within 10 she's saying that she wants to die.

She's only happy if I am sitting with her explaining over and over to her why she is here.

First I show her a picture of her and Dad sitting in front of their house. Then I explain that Dad died. When her face falls I say that he was ready and it would be wrong to call him back. She nods her head wisely and says she understands.

'Then', I say, 'I suggested that you come to live with me. I showed you this picture of our house (I show her the estate agent's blurb) and you agreed it would be fun. You've lived here happily for four years now.'

'Four years?!' she says at this point, 'then why don't I remember?' 'Because', I say, 'you've had a nasty infection that has made you feel rotten. But you're getting better now. Soon you'll feel fine.'

This story calms her. It's not entirely true, of course. For a start I have no idea whether she has a urine infection. Neither has anyone else.

When the doctor came she wouldn't let him touch her. When he tried she growled at him. The district nurse got as far as trying to take a blood sample. But the minute Mum felt the needle she screamed blue murder. The nurse and I backed off double quick. We didn't even try to get a urine sample.

We're going to treat her 'blind' with antibiotics. Mum has never had problems with antibiotics, so even if there is no infection she shouldn't react badly. If an infection is part of the problem they'll help clear it up.

My days are agony. One minute I feel huge compassion. The next I feel murderous. Mostly I feel helpless. How can you help someone who has no memory at all?

Only by giving them your full attention.

But I simply can't do it. Not only because I am so busy, but also because it's not in my nature.

Tomorrow my sister is coming for a week whilst I go walking in the Lake District. When I get back I will rethink the care situation sensibly.

So think of me next week striding across the hills, free as a bird!

The University of Stirling has done a lot of research on designing homes to maximize the comfort and minimize the confusion of those with dementia. The result is published in three books (and a useful checklist) – see details under Miscellaneous in the Resources chapter, pages 275–84.

Tether's End

So much for my holiday. Three days back and it's as if I haven't been away.

Before I went I had a dreadful week trying to stabilize Mum. She was constantly on my heels, bad-tempered and uncharacteristically aggressive. I was drained, near screaming pitch and desperately conscious of the work I wasn't doing. I couldn't wait for my sister to arrive.

But when she did we had a hissing, spitting row. Not surprising, perhaps. She had had an exhausting five-hour journey, and was expecting me to be sociable. But I was desperate to shut myself in my study and tackle some of the backlog so I could go with a clear conscience.

We made up over a pizza after Mum went to bed. Then I worked until 2 a.m., got up at 5 a.m. and cleared the most guilt-making stuff. I was also able to work on the train.

But a huge amount of resentment is building up. I feel my life isn't my own, and that all I do is think of other people.

In order to go away I have to rely on the goodwill of others. This puts me in the position of supplicant, which I loathe. It also makes me responsible for their comfort.

So I make up their beds, remember their likes and dislikes as I shop, empty drawers for them, order their paper and try to write down everything they might need to know while they are here (chiropodist Tuesday, bins Wednesday …). And so on.

All this might seem straightforward, and so it is when Mum is her normal self and I am on top of things. But when she's as she currently is it can feel like the final straw. My head feels as if it might explode with all the things I have to do.

It's not that I am not grateful. But to be honest I am sick of being grateful. And I am sick of thinking of other people. The person I need to think about is *me*.

I am unable to sleep (partly thanks to Mum), and stressed out by Mum's looking miserable and following me around, and by the work that I'm not doing. When Mum's at day care I can't stop crying.

Yesterday I rang the doctor. I burst into tears as he came on the phone, so I think he's got the message. He arranged for the Community Psychiatric Nurse to ring.

'What do you need?' she asked. 'Help,' I said. 'What sort of help?' she asked, quite reasonably. But I can't answer that. Everywhere I look I see contradictions. Mum needs me, but I have nothing left.

What I need is for her to die peacefully in her sleep, dreaming of Daddy and the cat.

> If the stress is rising, don't ignore it. In this situation you are your first priority. Carve out two hours. Spend one somewhere beautiful, preferably in the fresh air. Then brainstorm your stress by answering two questions: What is stressing you? What would help? Whatever you learn, act on it. You'll note I didn't do this. More fool me.

The Future

Things are getting back to normal. The antibiotics, plus the one-to-one care I have been giving Mum, are working. She is smiling, joking and much more relaxed. The virago of the last few weeks is no more.

But it was *exhausting*. I am a worn-out rag, and my week's holiday is a distant memory (what would it have been like if I hadn't had it, though?). I am now tackling the huge backlog of work that has built up. But I must find time to think about the future.

That things can get so scary so quickly is extremely worrying. I can't take many more months like the last. When Mum is herself, caring for her is a doddle ... well, a doddle compared to when she isn't herself. She's so cheerful and good-natured that I *want* to do things for her – it feels easy even if it isn't.

But I am obviously a fair-weather carer. When she's as she has been recently, caring is a nightmare. Mum treated me as an enemy, as someone she needed to fight, someone who wanted to hurt her. It was truly dreadful.

It is humbling to realize that many carers deal with this all the time. I don't know how they manage. No one cares in order to be appreciated, but not being appreciated – indeed, being treated as a threat, is just the pits. It wouldn't be human not to ask why one is bothering.

Good question, that. Why does one bother? It would be much easier to shuffle people into a home, where they'd be out of sight and out of mind. So many people seem to think this is the obvious answer that I think they think I am a mug for looking after Mum.

As I see it I have three options: (1) I implement – less clumsily – the care package made possible by the Direct Payments, (2) I get a live-in carer, or (3) I find a home.

The first is beginning to seem reasonable now Mum is back to normal. Two weeks ago it seemed impossible given Mum's distraught state.

The second would mean my home really *wouldn't* be my own. And I'd lose my study so the carer could have somewhere to sleep.

The third ... well, the third. Could I put Mum in a home? I have been allowing myself, tentatively, mentally, to explore the freedom it would give me, but it feels dangerous. I know my own capacity for guilt, especially where Mum is concerned.

But I am only 52, and I have a life to live. So far I have lived it as well as caring for Mum. But can this continue?

I should be interested in your advice ...

> I wrote this soon after my friend Philippa's husband had gone into a home. She gave me a good telling-off for the phrase 'shuffle people into a home'. 'For many people', she said, 'putting people into a home is an ignominious defeat. It's the last thing they want to do.' I discovered this for myself later. If I've upset you with this phrase, I am sorry.

Back with a Vengeance

Things were improving last week. This week Mum is back to normal with a vengeance.

Every morning she has got up without protest – a miracle! She has had two or three baths with minimal grumbling. Today I cut and cleaned her fingernails without her screaming once (she does a good scream, my mum, usually when the clippers are nowhere near her actual nails).

It's as if she is so relieved that her routine is back that she loves the whole world.

It can be embarrassing. Last night we were taken for tea with someone who might provide Mum with an 'adult placement'. This is a substitute for respite care which, you may remember, did not go smoothly for Mum.

In an adult placement a family or, in this case, a single person, will have Mum to stay for the odd weekend, a day here or there, or even a full week.

For me this would be fantastic. It would enable me to have time in my own home on my own. I really suffer from never feeling my home is my own, and it would be marvellous to have people to lunch or supper, or to lounge around reading the paper, or to laze in a bath without Mum's coming to find me. I might even get to read a book.

Jill, who organizes adult placement, collected us at 4. Mum greeted her like the prodigal daughter: 'How *very* nice to see you!' she said, throwing her arms around an astonished Jill and kissing her enthusiastically, 'You look wonderful!'

They have met before. Once.

But this was nothing to the way Mum greeted Sandy [all names have been changed], the person who might provide placement. As soon as she opened the door, Mum smothered her with kisses, gripped her hand and told her about ten times that she liked her very much.

Phyllis, aged 96, and on placement with Sandy, was dozing in a chair. At least she was until Mum grasped her to her bosom and told her she had beautiful hair. I don't know when Phyllis was last told this, but her smile was something to behold (even more toothless than Mum's).

We were shown around the house, with Mum exclaiming every second about the beauty of this and that, the wonder of that and this and the sheer marvellousness of Sandy and everyone else. She kept grabbing my hand and giving me a smacking kiss.

I wasn't sure whether to apologize for Mum's exuberance, or act as if she was like this all the time. Sandy seemed to like it, but the proof will be if she's willing to take Mum on.

Keep your fingers crossed for me …

Adult placement didn't work for us. The first time we went Sandy had forgotten we were coming and gone out. I had taken a day off work, booked the Octobus (a superb and very cheap service for disabled and elderly people) and was looking forward enormously to an afternoon off. It was devastating.

Money Money Money

Money! It's always a problem isn't it? It's not usually, though, a case of having too much. But currently that's my problem.

It started when the Council granted me Direct Payments backdated to 2nd November. Since being told I would be getting them I hadn't dared actually spend anything. Well, would *you* have believed it?

But there it was – nearly £6,000, representing £403 per week for some months.

But I have now taken on board the strings it comes with.

I only get that amount, for example, if I use agency care. If I use private carers the amount is reduced to just over £200 a week. This means I can only pay private carers about £8 an hour. This is reasonable, but far from riches.

If I use private carers I must become an employer. This involves my having to pay tax and National Insurance for the carer. It also involves contracts, official paid holidays, health and safety, and employers' insurance. I am assured all this is simple, but it is nevertheless daunting (and I really don't need more to do).

A particular nuisance is that I can't pay relatives' expenses without having to pay tax and National Insurance on them. If my sister drives from Leeds, for example, and I pay her petrol, then I must declare her 'earnings' to the Inland Revenue and complete numerous forms.

As she's retired she doesn't even have to pay this tax. But to get it back she must also complete numerous forms. What a palaver.

Then there's the fact that the money can only be used for Mum's care. I think this means that I can't use it for a cleaner. Yet this would be seriously useful – as Mum's incontinence gets worse I am constantly cleaning, but I never have time to do things like vacuum the sitting room, dust the bookshelves or wash the kitchen floor.

Finally, if I do not use the money, it gets clawed back. So I might lose all the money that built up before the first payment arrived. I might even lose the money that built up over the last few dreadful weeks when I've had to cancel care to get Mum stabilized.

One solution would be to go away for a couple of weeks. My goodness, how wonderful a proper break would be. But I can't do this before I have in place one or two carers Mum is happy with. She'd be happy with one of my brothers or my sister, of course, but they don't find it easy to get away at short notice.

Still, as problems go, it's one I'd far rather have than some others I can think of!

> Incontinence. You'll get used to it. I kept spray disinfectant in every loo (the apple-smelling ones are nice). I bought industrial-sized quantities of latex gloves (but usually didn't have time to put them on). Disposable pants are a godsend. Your best incontinence aid is a sense of humour.

Angelic Choir

When I retire I intend to join a choir. The Bach Choir would be wonderful – just imagine singing the St Matthew Passion – but they require the ability to sight-read. Perhaps I should learn to sight-read, then join a choir?

I love to sing and have, I like to think, a reasonable voice. This is from Mum. Dad was completely tone deaf.

This didn't stop him singing. He used to make up songs for us. The one I remember most went: 'Come o'er the stream Richard, sweet Richard, sweet Richard, come o'er the stream,

Richard and play with Marianne.' This went on for as many verses as Dad could bear, and Richard and I adored it.

But if Mum were in the house Dad would manage only the opening bar. Mum would instantly appear, screeching 'Phil, please! Stop that dreadful noise. I can't bear it.'

We thought she was a spoilsport. If Dad were in a wicked mood, we'd egg him on. He'd wait until Mum closed the door and start up again.

Mum had – indeed, has – a wonderful voice. I loved standing beside her in church as she sang. I was proud of her, and sorry for the children whose mothers had run-of-the-mill voices.

When Mum retired, and before she developed Alzheimer's, she joined the choir at the local church. She adored the camaraderie of weekly choir practice and the Sunday services.

She particularly enjoyed singing at weddings. This wasn't only because of the £5 she was paid, though that was a major incentive, it was also because she was a sucker for weddings. Every bride was the most beautiful she'd ever seen, every groom the 'dishiest' (Mum's slang was always at least 20 years out of date).

As the Alzheimer's started to bite, Mum's presence at choir practice became a rarity, her contribution to Sunday services – er – patchy. She still loved a wedding, but only a brave bride would rely on her.

To their great credit, however, the choir kept her on. More. They would ring to remind her about choir practice, offer her lifts on Sunday, and they continued to pay her for weddings long after her timing had gone and they had to sing EXTREMELY LOUDLY to drown her out.

This was characteristic of her church. They were wonderful. I don't think anyone ever gave the impression that the effort required to maintain her status as parishioner or chorister was a burden.

Mum has given up going to church. But she still sings. What she sings bears little resemblance to whatever she is singing along to, but sing along she does. Lustily.

I still get pleasure from listening to her.

> People with dementia can sometimes be frightened by their own reflection in a mirror (or even the glass of a picture). It might be best to take down larger mirrors, and certainly those in your piglet's room.

Getting Up

Mum did not want to get up this morning. 'Poor you,' I commiserated as I yanked open the curtains. 'I didn't want to get up either.' 'But' I said as I pulled off her duvet, 'I've got to go to work: you'd *hate* to be on your own for seven hours.'

There's no way I'd really leave Mum on her own for seven hours, or even seven minutes. But the threat worked and, still groaning, she allowed me to dress her.

But I do feel sorry for her. We all know the horrors of heaving ourselves out of a warm bed, especially on a day like today when the wind is howling fit to bust. I also remember how ghastly *I* was when Mum had to get *me* up.

At first I moaned and groaned as impotently as Mum does now. But then I got clever. I am rather ashamed to admit what I did. But it worked.

I would set my alarm for some dreadful time like 4 a.m. When it went off I would noisily trip to the loo and spend some time in there, groaning every now and then, and making sure the whole house knew where I was.

Then I would brush my teeth and go and tell Mum I felt dreadful.

Mum just wanted to go back to sleep herself, of course. She would wake up just enough to establish I wasn't dying, then she'd tuck me back in bed, telling me to try to sleep.

This I did very successfully. In the morning, though, you would think I hadn't slept a wink, so sick had I been.

I know Mum suspected me of lead-swinging. But in the morning rush she would often just give up. It must have seemed a great deal easier just to leave me, especially as she couldn't be certain I wasn't ill.

I would then have a delightful duvet day, reading, raiding the larder and trying out her make-up.

Naturally by the end of the working day I was back in bed claiming to feel slightly better, but not at all sure I'd be ready for school in the morning.

Dad had more of the measure of me. He'd burst into the room singing 'Wakey, wakey! Rise and shine! Shake a leg!' He'd have the curtains open and the blankets off me before I knew what was happening.

Dad, of course, would have been up for hours, lighting the fires, getting the Rayburn going and making sure there was enough hot water. In those days we had to scrape the ice off the inside of the windows in the morning.

Mum was once as devious as I was. Thank goodness for small mercies.

Piglets often feel the cold cruelly. When the heating needs to be on, put all their clothes, especially their underwear and socks, onto the radiators for a good 5 minutes before you start dressing them. Mum used to sigh with pleasure as she put on a toasty vest.

Interviews

I have spent the week interviewing carers. Last week I fielded application forms, and the week before, telephone calls in response to my advertisement. Anyone would think I had nothing to do other than think about Mum's care.

But if I find a carer who does the trick it will be worth it.

I already have a carer without whom I could not cope. Anita started as a part-time secretary, but she was soon putting more time into Mum and the secretarial stuff fell by the wayside.

Anita is Croatian, she has a PhD in philosophy and qualified as a nurse during the war in Croatia in the 1990s. She stands on no ceremony with me, telling me off for leaving lights on and for failing to recycle things properly.

She teases Mum and takes no nonsense, but Mum seems happy to put up with it. Mum seems to *enjoy* it. Anita can even give Mum a bath.

Anita is a complete star.

One of Anita's key charms, certainly for Mum, is her two-year-old son, Andrej. Andrej is a delight. He is the opposite of shy, and he adores Mum. I encourage Anita to bring Andrej whenever she wants.

When they arrive, Andrej darts in crying 'Lesley? Lesley? Where is Lesley?' If Mum is still in bed or at day care, he keeps asking for her until she arrives. Then the two of them collude in driving Anita completely mad.

They are exhausting. Last time they were together they found a squeaky toy mouse, discarded by the cats (far too grand to play with toys). Mum and Andrej were tossing this mouse between them with gay abandon and screams of delight.

As I left it seemed unlikely Anita was going to get either of them to bed for hours. But she was still smiling.

I have tried to persuade Anita to leave her husband and move in (sorry, Sinisa). But she's not having it. So I need another carer for when Anita is on holiday or can't do a shift.

My advertisement attracted lots of replies. A few of them I didn't take to the application stage: if I couldn't understand them, how were they going to work with Mum? Many to whom I sent a form didn't return it: advanced Alzheimer's deters even professional carers.

But I have been pleased by those I have interviewed. There are some really nice people around. Often they are people who started to care for a family member, discovered they were good at it and got a lot out of it, and have continued.

With any luck I might be able to report next week that I have found someone who has a chance of being a second Anita.

At this time Anita was trying to have a second baby (the gorgeous Uma arrived18 months later). I was supporting this and kept my fingers crossed for her. This is evidence of my ignorance of the implications of Direct Payments. Had Anita succeeded in getting pregnant whilst she was caring for Mum, I'd have had to pay maternity leave. AAArgh!

Handkerchief

'My innards appear to have gone into my long ones' complained Mum yesterday.

Hm. Mum's loss of language adds to the gaiety of days. This gem meant her handkerchief had gone too far up her sleeve.

Mum's handkerchiefs are the bane of my life. If she doesn't have a handkerchief she will – quite unconsciously – make everyone's life a misery.

The search starts at her wrists. Pulling her sleeve out, she peers in. Then she starts rummaging. Then she'll try the other wrist. Then, snuffling in earnest, she'll widen her search to her armpits and her bra.

Then her pockets. She'll turn them all inside out v e r y s l o w l y.

Then she'll turn to her waistband and her knickers.

If no handkerchief appears, she'll use something else. Napkins are wonderful. Loo paper will do (she takes a whole ribbon, then puts it in her pocket. It *always* ends up in the washing machine). But failing these she'll use blankets, tea towels or whatever might be to hand.

I have bought her so many handkerchiefs I am single-handedly keeping the industry alive. She has two drawers' full. Great man-sized things.

I keep handkerchiefs in every room. But it doesn't matter how many she starts out with, she will soon have lost them all. At night she must have one under each pillow and one in her breast pocket.

After use, Mum follows a painful (to me) ritual: the hand-kerchief must be folded and put away.

Simple enough, you might think. But not for Mum. The folding, for example, is an art form. It takes ages and clearly matters a great deal.

First she lays the handkerchief flat on her lap. She then folds it in half. The corners must meet exactly. If whoever ironed it (usually Mum herself) hasn't flattened the corners, this will cause great anxiety. Each fold must be the same size as the last, and the whole must then be secured in some way.

I am used to having a bundle of handkerchief thrust at me so that I can secure it. I have found the best thing to do is exclaim at the neatness of the bundle, and to suggest Mum put it safely in her sleeve so she'll know where it is next time.

It is fun to watch visitors seeing Mum's handkerchief ritual for the first time. Initially they look puzzled, then distressed as it sinks in that this is a manifestation of the Alzheimer's. But they soon get used to it.

I have no idea where the ritual came from. It started ages ago. But in some odd way it makes her less anxious.

That's got to be worth something.

As your life swooshes past in a haze of crises, meals, appointments, washing cycles, 'little accidents', temper tantrums and alarums from the day care centre, try consciously to set aside time to do something you enjoy with your piglet. When they're gone, it's these times you'll remember.

Knickers

It is time to discuss a delicate subject: the matter of knickers.

For the last three years Mum and I have managed successfully with paper knickers. These look and feel just like ordinary knickers. But they can be disposed of without fuss.

I have no idea what the disposal of them is doing to our carbon footprint. I can't say I care very much. Anyway, every time I dispose of a pair I reuse a plastic bag. But the paper knicker solution is no longer working.

The trouble with the knicker problem is that it is inextricably linked to the dignity problem.

You imagine how you'd feel if a middle-aged woman whom you *think* you know, but you wouldn't swear to it, followed you into the loo and told you to take your trousers off.

Like Mum, you'd probably say 'But I don't *want* my trousers off!' or '*Why* should I take my trousers off?' Then, blow you down if she doesn't want your knickers off too!

It would *not* help to be told that you need to be washed and changed. *Outrageous!* Who does she think you are: a two-year-old?

Poor Mum gets subjected to this indignity at least twice a day. It's amazing that she ever does it without complaint.

Sometimes, though, she completely refuses. Then I wait until she is sitting on the loo and try to pull them off.

This results in an unseemly tug of war. Sometimes I find myself on my back on the floor with her trousers in my hands. Other times Mum wins, and ends up waving her still-trousered legs in the air.

This doesn't leave either of us feeling very dignified.

Lately, though, Mum has needed to be changed more often. The people at Willows have mentioned it. They have also, on a couple of occasions, sent her home wearing a sort of padded thong. Not quite a thong, because the stringy bits are at the sides. But it looks almost as uncomfortable.

At our recent care review it was suggested that I might like to discuss the problem with the district nurse. As I was seeing the doctor, however, I mentioned it to him. He talked about our getting some knickers with a sort of 'trapdoor'.

Don't you just love these technical terms?

Trapdoor knickers would enable Mum to be changed without her having to take the rest of her clothes off. That sounds good. So I checked out the catalogue. But I could only find the thongs, plus various garments that probably make sense once you know how to use them.

Goodness, though, I am extremely glad Mum is not male!

There are manufacturers of disposable pants who make express deliveries to your door the day after you call them. You may think you'll never run out of pants, but believe me, one day you will. Good to have the phone number of such people to hand (I used HDS, who were brilliant – see the Resources chapter, pages 275–84).

Time-wasting

What a week. Well, fortnight really. I have mentioned the Direct Payments I am now getting and the HUGE administrative burden that comes with them. It is possible that the burden of time-wasting is even worse.

The Council has taken on an organization whose task it is to explain Direct Payments, and to administer them, if that is what the carer wants. It seemed to be worth at least a meeting. So I set up an appointment.

The young woman who came seemed a nice person. But it quickly became clear she knew virtually nothing about Direct Payments. The hour I spent with her was an exercise in trying to keep my temper whilst she told me loads of things I already knew.

Every time I asked her a question she merely repeated what she had already told me. Incredibly, I started to feel *sorry* for her. Hardly her fault if she hadn't been properly trained.

The upshot of the meeting was that I must insure myself in case a carer breaks her leg and sues me, and I must register as a small employer with the Inland Revenue. She gave me a lot of telephone numbers and off she went.

I spoke to a nice man at the insurance company and we started to complete the form so I'd get immediate cover.

Things went pear-shaped almost immediately. The nice young woman had impressed on me that the insurance should be in Mum's name, as she was the one getting the Direct Payments. The man I was speaking to insisted the policy had to be in my name because I was the one employing the carers.

AAAArgh! There followed a merry-go-round of calls in which I was batted from one organization to the other, ending up near tears with frustration.

Trying to get registered as an employer was equally frustrating. I rang one of the numbers the nice young woman had given me. The person on the other end knew nothing of Direct Payments and was extremely unhelpful.

Another number yielded a lovely woman who also knew nothing about Direct Payments, but who offered to ring my nice young woman and clarify things. She came back with another number which led to a promise to send me a CD Rom. (Oh joy.) This has yet to arrive.

So have I succeeded in registering myself as a small employer? I have no idea.

In the meantime, one of my new carers, Carol, is turning out to be just incredible. She is with Mum in the kitchen now. They are making a chocolate cake (gluten-free, of course) and chatting away as if they have known each other for years.

At least I know it'll all be worth it.

> If there are people in and out of your house all the time, get a 'key safe'. It attaches to the wall, your key is kept inside and you can give the combination to anyone who needs it. Saves giving them all keys, and you can change the combination any time.

Spontaneity

My life is transformed. Suddenly I am almost a free agent. I can say 'yes' to invitations. I can do a full day's work. I can do *spontaneous*. These Direct Payments are marvellous!

Tonight a friend is unexpectedly in town. He suggested we meet for an early supper before he goes back to London.

Two months ago I would have had to embark on a ring-round to find someone willing to Mum-sit. More likely, knowing the ghastliness of doing this (and the slim chances of success), I would have said 'no'.

I was saying 'no' to a lot of invitations: *not* the way to avoid resentment.

Now, though, I can ring Carol or Anita and, so long as one or the other is free, I am off! Even if they're not free I have other strings to my bow – money can undoubtedly buy some sorts of happiness.

I have a feeling this has come in the nick of time. Mum really is deteriorating. Yesterday, for example, we were hanging out the washing. Two months ago she would have done it competently, albeit slowly, on her own. Yesterday she wasn't sure what the pegs were for.

First she tried to attach a towel to the line without a peg. When I gave her a peg, she attached it to the line without the towel. When I demonstrated the use of the peg to attach the towel to the line she just didn't get it.

But she knows she's not getting it. And she obviously feels defensive. We all know and so, apparently, does Mum, that the best form of defence is attack.

I find myself under attack often these days.

I ask Mum if she wants to finish the cereal she's obviously forgotten, for example, and she'll round on me: 'I *am* finishing it,' she'll say indignantly, 'leave me alone.' Or if I make her get up after she's got into bed with all her clothes on, she accuses me of persecuting her.

These are not the jokey complaints she used to make. These are the heartfelt complaints of one who feels she is being made to do something she doesn't see the point of.

Mum doesn't go to day care on Sunday or Monday. Until recently I have been on duty day and night for 48 hours. It is very isolating to be with someone who thinks you're constantly getting at them. Especially when you're actually trying to help. By Monday evening I have been at screaming pitch.

But now I can afford someone to relieve me for a few hours: I can go swimming or walking or I can shut myself in my bedroom to read a book …

Luxury!

Hm. It *was* wonderful having the money to buy in care. If I had had it early enough it might have enabled me to care for Mum through to the end. But perhaps I am being unfair? Mum was deteriorating significantly. Perhaps it was this, rather than the administration associated with Direct Payments, that was making life so difficult?

Place-blindness

Whenever Mum and I socialize with people who don't know Mum, their first question is always: 'Do you live around here?'

This means that Mum is stumped right away. She has no idea where she lives. Or where she is. Or where she's been. All she knows is that she is here (with no idea where 'here' is).

You might think this is the Alzheimer's. But Mum never did have a sense of place. I always thought this a touching sign of self-esteem: I am here, nothing else matters. But this might be because I share Mum's place-blindness.

This handicap has never bothered us. We always had fun together wherever we were going. We used to talk and laugh so much that, when finally we wondered where we were, we'd discover we were miles out of our way, often completely lost.

One day we went walking in Alderley Edge, a beautiful spot near where Mum used to live. We were talking about life, the universe and everything, until we suddenly realized it was getting dark and we had no idea where we were.

When I say 'no idea', I really mean *no idea*. We didn't even know in which direction the car was. It was really rather nasty. We managed to keep cheerful by talking of the cave we'd sleep in. But we were hugely relieved to find the car just as darkness fell in earnest.

Then there was the occasion we set off for IKEA in, I think, Warrington. Anyway, somewhere neither of us knew, but near enough, we thought, to make the drive worthwhile.

Well, it probably was reasonably near. But again we got talking and again we found ourselves lost. This time in far less pleasant surroundings. We were on a motorway and, we thought, going in the wrong direction. We found our way off it, got back on and then found we really *were* going in the wrong direction. Too late. We were stuck for miles.

We got to IKEA. But it was closed.

Mobile phones now make it impossible to get comprehensively lost. I recently cycled to Woodstock with a friend. This usually takes 50 minutes. An hour and a half in, therefore, I realized something was wrong.

My sister, when I used my mobile to ask where we were, hooted with laughter. Judy has a most un-Talbot-like feel for where she is. My friend, who had thought I knew where I was going, looked on in bemusement.

But mobiles came too late for Mum. Anyway, she enjoyed getting lost. She claimed she met some of the nicest people when she asked for directions.

But people always fell over themselves to help Mum. They still do.

I wish Mum's Alzheimer's had held off until e-mail came in. She would have *adored* it. She must have been one of the first ordinary people to get a computer. She took to it straight away (though only as a word processor). Mum was a communicator extraordinaire – e-mail would have struck her as completely magical.

Another Loss

Mum has always adored children. Show her a picture of a baby and she goes all soft and squidgy. Let her, whilst out, see a pushchair and there's no stopping her until we have inspected the child, ahh'd and cooed, prodded it in the tummy and congratulated its mother or father on its beauty.

Until recently, this suited everyone. The parent of the child beams, the child gurgles and Mum goes on her way feeling all's right with the world. It makes me feel good, too: how lucky I am to have such a mum.

But this happy state of affairs is coming to an end. As the Alzheimer's closes in, Mum's instincts with children are deserting her. She has started to frighten them.

First her behaviour became an unthinking expression of her adoration. Spotting a child, she would swoop on it with cries of delight, tickling it as if it were her own, giving it bear hugs and play-biting its neck. Often the child had no warning at all. Especially if Mum swooped from behind.

The resulting cacophony brings parents running from everywhere. I have to disentangle Mum from the screaming child, trying, red-faced, to explain whilst leaving Mum with as much dignity as possible.

To their great credit, most parents, after the initial shock, have been understanding. No one has suggested to me that Mum shouldn't be allowed out. All have assured me that the child will be fine. But I do worry. Of course I worry. Both for Mum's equilibrium, and for the child and the way it will interact in future with the elderly.

Very young children seem to adore the elderly. But once children reach school age they start to shy away from the old, sometimes in a hurtful way. I wonder why this is. It can't always be the case that when they were younger they met someone like Mum in a supermarket. Perhaps they get tainted with society's negative view of the very old? Perhaps they just become too self-conscious?

These days, however, it is not only older children who are wary of Mum. Even her darling Andrej has started to back off.

Mum herself has become self-conscious. How is it that despite her lack of memory and language, despite her confusion, she is still so sensitive to others' responses to her? In an almost lucid moment recently she said to me, of Andrej, 'He doesn't like me any more.'

She is probably right. It makes me want to weep.

Both Carers UK and the Princess Royal Trust for Carers do marvellous fact sheets. These explain very simply exactly what you need to know about a given topic. They cover just about anything a carer might want to know about caring. Contact details in the Resources chapter (pages 275–84).

Entertainment

My goodness, I have had a *terrible* morning.

Mum now can't do anything independently. Either I have to steel myself to her looking miserably into space, or entertain her.

The space-staring makes me feel agitated and guilty. Soon I start saying things like 'Why don't you *do* something?' Then Mum gets agitated and guilty. Not a recipe for relaxation.

If I am extremely busy I grit my teeth to the space-staring. But trying to work out PAYE, write letters or compose e-mails with Mum staring glumly at me is extremely difficult.

Sometimes Mum *wants* to be entertained. She'll pull my hand, plonk herself next to me and complain every five seconds about having nothing to do.

I used to be able to leave Mum staring into space and work elsewhere. But, these days, the minute I'm out of sight she'll come to find me.

If Mum wants to be entertained, therefore, the only thing I can do is entertain her.

But this means giving her my undivided attention. I can't just give her a book, I have to read it with her. Not *to* her but *with* her. She isn't a child, after all, and she gets irritated if I imply – however accurately – that she can't read herself.

Nor can I do domestic chores and expect her to sit and watch: she must help. As you might imagine, Mum's 'helping' is not helpful. She needs constant supervision, and she needs to be 'talked through' everything.

And the talking she wants is not the talking I would do if I were thinking aloud.

That would go: 'Oh, God, when am I ever going to be able to do this or that?' or 'I *wish* she'd leave me alone for a minute' or 'If only I could get this finished' or 'If she says that one more time, I'll scream.'

But the life-saver (from my point of view) is that Mum is a brilliant sleeper. On Sundays and Mondays, when she doesn't go to day care, she'll often stay in bed until 2 p.m. This enables me to get some work done so that by the afternoon I am more relaxed about entertaining her.

Today is Monday. I was expecting a morning to myself and an afternoon of entertaining Mum. But Mum got up at 8. AARGH!

So I got on the phone immediately. Some aspects of the Direct Payments are wonderful. Within the hour, Carol was here. First they made a soup and sang songs. Now they are walking round the garden laughing together. In an hour's time Anita will take over.

All I have to do now is calm down so I can get some work done.

The entertainment problem is a major one. At this point even the professional carers were finding it difficult. I suspect that this might be the point at which to seriously consider a nursing home. The good homes are set up with the entertainment of people with dementia at least partly in mind.

Appetite

Life is fraught. Mum's deterioration is moving so fast I can hardly keep up. For months, years even, she stayed reasonably stable (although others noticed her deterioration). But at the moment she is sinking faster and faster.

For the first time, too, she is physically deteriorating. She used to be extremely – er – robust. But she has lost a huge amount of weight. Her clothes are hanging off her. As I helped her out of the bath yesterday I noticed the tops of her arms are beginning to look skeletal.

Skeletal? Mum?

Mum has always had a huge appetite. She *adored* her food. I have fond memories (and a photograph she loathed) of her looking hungrily at the largest knickerbocker glory you ever saw. She polished it off in minutes. Wanting to treat herself, she used to drive herself to the nearest Little Chef and order three portions of their garlic mushrooms. Appetite has never been a problem for Mum.

About six months ago, though, she started to find it difficult to eat. I began cutting up her food. That worked for a while. But she continued to find the knife and fork difficult. I substituted a spoon and fork. Then I removed the fork.

Last night she was trying to eat with the spoon the wrong way up.

All my healthy eating rules have gone out of the window. I now cook whatever I think might tempt Mum. Last week I fried some potatoes for her. I have never fried potatoes in my life!

Not only that, I served them with a mushroom omelette fried in butter, and covered the lot with tomato sauce. I felt strangely proud when she ate the lot.

But 'the lot' was about half the amount she would have eaten before.

Her teeth are part of the problem. Last time she lost her dentures I decided it wasn't worth replacing them. She'd had the pair she lost only about three weeks. They cost £450.

So Mum has one tooth in front at the top. But she still has enough at the back to be able to chew. But apples – which Mum used to eat continuously – have become virtually impossible.

I wonder whether her teeth are hurting her? I have made a dental appointment, but am dreading it. Mum is not going to take kindly to someone poking around in her mouth.

But last night was something new: I am not sure, but I suspect Mum wasn't even sure that her food was for eating. I had to help her, spoonful by spoonful.

To think Mum might need feeding is the most daunting thing I have yet faced.

Your piglet may be able to feed themselves for longer if you buy a set of large colourful cutlery with rubber handles.
Use plain crockery, too. Vivid patterns can leave your piglet forlornly scraping up the 'spinach' or 'soup' that is in fact a painted rose bush or clematis-covered trellis.

Manipulation

'Go away,' Mum hissed 'I just want to die.'

All I was doing was trying to get her to go back upstairs to get dressed.

Mum has been uncharacteristically manipulative lately. She has started to claim that she wants to die fairly frequently. It is clearly a sign of her being unhappy, but is it really a sign that she wants to die? I don't think so. I think that what she wants is for life to go back to normal.

She wants to be able to communicate, for example. At the moment, whenever she tries to say something it comes out all wrong. The only clue to her meaning is the context, and often that is not enough.

She also wants to be able to enjoy her food. But when she tries to eat she misses her mouth. Or she crams so much in that she's in danger of choking.

She also wants to be alone with me, knowing where she is and why. But there's no way I can cope on my own any more. So, instead of our nice cosy routine, the house is always full of people coming and going.

It must be a nightmare for her.

So much so, in fact, that I am beginning to think that she is no longer benefiting from living with me. This feeling became so strong last week that I actually went to see a home that someone recommended.

I wasn't expecting much. But I liked it. The rooms were nice and light. There was a conservatory in which a group of ladies were sitting 'talking' to some carers. There was a large television on the wall. It was switched off. Good.

Even better, they said they would be prepared for Mum to come to lunch a few times to see how she managed. I shall certainly take them up on that.

But I find myself thinking, 'If only I could go into her room one morning to find that she had died peacefully in her sleep.' It would feel so right for her to die whilst she's still living with me, and before this deterioration gets worse.

Already she is becoming a different person. Occasionally I can still see Mum, but mostly Mum has been replaced by this bad-tempered, manipulative old woman who spends her life complaining, and expecting me to run after her.

The other day, after several hours of fetching her this and that, finding her stuff to do and trying to get her interested in something, I found that she was using a handful of my Spring bulbs as a bookmark.

I really hated her at that moment.

I'm now sure that Mum should already have been in a nursing home at this point. After this blog, a reader suggested I take seriously Mum's claim that she wanted to die. So difficult, though. After all, what could I have done? I was so relieved when she went into her home and reverted to her normal cheerful self.

In the Way

Oh, dear. The Direct Payments I thought were so marvellous might prove to be the final straw.

I am good with money. I was Dad's Receiver for years. I have had Mum's Power of Attorney for even longer. Yet it took me three days to understand PAYE.

The Inland Revenue helpline is wonderful (especially Mary Spiers. Thank you, Mary.) But there are so many ifs and buts, and so much misleading information (mainly from Social Services).

Since 2nd November 2007 I have been paying Anita as self-employed. I was told that was fine. But it's not. Now I have to work out how much tax and National Insurance Anita should have paid, and claw it back. I must also pay my contribution.

I haven't screwed up the courage even to look at this.

Then, as none of my carers can work regular hours, I must negotiate a new rota each week. First I ask one what she can do. Then I ring the other. Then I renegotiate with the first. Each week there's a different pattern to my own week as I fill different gaps.

But my life was packed to the gills before starting Direct Payments. I have never been so far behind with so many deadlines: I am constantly nagged by guilt.

I am also constantly in the way.

At 8.30 a carer arrives. So I must either be out or hiding in the study. Then I can't return, or I must keep out of the way, until 6. My home is not my own.

Nor do I have a workplace to go to. I (supposedly) work from home. In fact I work from a café in town. I used to enjoy this. It was a break from being at home and the bustle helped me concentrate. But now I'm there for 8 hours. Too fattening. Too expensive.

I tried the library but kept ending up next to people with a sniffing habit (aaargh!).

The domestic chores used to be a pleasant way of punctuating my working day. Now I have to do them during the evening or at weekends. But then Mum has to 'help'. Or I have to do them before Mum gets up or after she has gone to bed.

I am so *tired*. Actually the word 'tired' doesn't do it. I am completely and utterly exhausted. I have no downtime. Everything revolves around Mum and her needs. My needs don't get a look-in.

But nor, now, do I feel I am *needed*.

'Nonsense!' you might say. But what Mum needs now is stability and constant care. Whom she gets it from is irrelevant so long as they are kind.

Mum is no longer getting any benefit from the fact that her main carer is *me*.

If you are in, or nearing, this position, please, please reconsider your objections to a nursing home. There are some very good ones around. Mum's nursing home, when she finally went into it, gave her a new lease of life. When I saw how happy she was it gave me my life back. Surely it's worth a try?

Equilibrium

The night before last Mum and I sobbed in each other's arms. She kept apologizing because I had to look after her, and I kept insisting it was a privilege. I acknowledged there were times I wanted to throw her out of the window, but said I was sure she must have wanted to do this to me when I was little. She thought about this, laughed, and said 'That's true!'

We felt so 'connected' that I became convinced she was going to die in the night. I think I went a little mad.

I moved her mattress downstairs into the sitting room. I then moved another mattress from the spare room so I could hold her hand as she slept. She has been hallucinating the last week or two and has been frightened on her own at night. She liked this arrangement and kept saying, 'Thank you, thank you, I love you.'

This made me weep again.

In the middle of the night I woke to find her duvet wet through and thought 'Oh, my goodness, she's wet herself.' Oddly, nothing else seemed wet. Anyway, I whisked away her duvet and brought down the one from my bed.

Half an hour later the bedclothes were wet again. That's when I discovered the sitting-room ceiling was leaking.

I believe in God, but sometimes ...

By noon the goodwill of the previous evening was dissipating. Mum had become again the horrible old bag she has been lately, and I was realizing what a rod I was making for my own back.

Whilst Mum sat there making disparaging noises, I took everything back upstairs (I had to wait for Anita to get Mum's mattress back up – love must have given me superhuman strength the night before). I remade her bed, my bed *and* the spare bed, and vowed that I'd never do all that again.

But I probably will. It's such an emotional roller-coaster. I can swing from deep love and compassion one minute to almost pure hatred the next. It is playing havoc with my equilibrium.

Actually, I don't have much equilibrium.

Last week I was so sure I was going to kill Mum (or myself) that I rang our doctor and told him. He was wonderful. He rang

Judy (my sister) and ascertained she could take over. Then he rang Carol to make sure she could fill the gap. In the meantime I rang Joanna, who immediately offered her house as sanctuary, and Joelle, who picked me up and took me there. This is what friends are for.

Whilst I was away the Social Services machine whirred into action. The process for getting Mum into a home has started.

I feel wretched.

How well I remember the night described. I think I was going slightly mad. Why didn't I just sleep in Mum's bed with her? Or bring her into mine? Why did I take everything downstairs? The strange lucidity of our conversation really did convince me she was going to die. I think I was panicking.

Undertakers

'Have you thought which undertaker we'll use?' asked my older brother five minutes after he arrived.

This was just after I had read the 'Care Domains' file drafted by our district nurse. This is the document upon which funding for nursing homes turns. I read it aghast. Every word of it is true. But, oh dear, I just don't think of Mum like that.

Looking at it from the outside, it brings home why I am not managing. Mum hits 'priority' or 'severe' on just about every measure. She is aggressive, clingy, depressed and unable to do anything for herself.

But having made a couple of comments, I completed my bit by saying something about Mum as she *really* is. Or, perhaps more accurately, Mum as she used to be. She was (and sometimes is) such a lovely person. Warm, funny, sharp, caring, irreverent, honest …

She was a fantastic Mum. Not particularly maternal in the abstract, but fiercely protective of her own children. That didn't stop her neglecting us. But it was a benign neglect which enabled us to get on with our own lives. It certainly suited me. Mum always had projects on the go. She was always passionate about something or other. I am proud to be like her in this.

Not that we didn't have our problems.

She used to say that, from when I was about 10, she recognized that I was going my own way in life whatever she said, so she set out to support me. And support me she did. Not in a traditionally motherly way, perhaps, but in *her* way. For example, when I left home at 16 to live in a bedsit in London, Mum saw me off at the station. As I closed the train door, she handed me an envelope. It contained £5 and a note saying that if I ever needed to get home I should use it, that she loved me, and that whatever happened I should never be afraid to come home.

I am frightened about going on holiday. Will she die before I get back? I can't not go because she might not die, and then where would I be? I need time away.

That's why my brother is here. And my sister. My other brother is coming at the weekend. Mum won't know what's hit her.

They know I have started the process to get her into a home. They also know that I think she may be in her final weeks (she now weighs less than I do).

But no, I haven't yet thought about which undertaker we'll use.

> If a clinging habit is already in place, resolve to break it. Make appropriate arrangements for your piglet's care. As the carer comes in, out you go. No reassuring or promising to be back soon. Don't even say 'goodbye'. Let the carer in and go. In 5 minutes your piglet will have forgotten you.

France

I have just spent nine wonderful days in the south of France! I am tanned, relaxed and at least 5 lb heavier despite swimming 100 lengths of the (very small) pool every day.

I can't tell you how glad I am I went. I was so afraid Mum was going to die that I very nearly cancelled. But when – in trepidation – I rang from the train to see what the situation was, Judy (my sister) put me onto her. She said in her old strong cheerful voice: 'Hello Lou, have you had a nice holiday?'

Lou???

She hasn't called me 'Lou' for ages (it's short for 'Louise', my middle name, and was my parents' pet name for me). These days, because she can't remember my name, Mum doesn't call me anything much: to have her call me 'Lou' was FANTASTIC!!

I'm very glad I went for nine days. For the first two or three days I was on tenterhooks, expecting to have to hurtle back any minute. But the expected phone call didn't come. And the sun was so hot, the pool so clear and inviting, the food so good and the company so stimulating, that slowly I stopped worrying. For about five days I relaxed completely.

I didn't even think about Mum until I decided I had to make the phone call from the train. The call made me feel I'd been given a 'get out of jail free' card: not only a holiday but a cheerful mum!

Judy says she has no idea why Mum's mood improved so radically. It is clear that she devoted a lot of time to Mum's well-being, reading to her, singing with her, etc., so it could be that. I don't often have time to give Mum the attention she craves.

Nor, to be honest, have I the patience: even if I didn't have to work I doubt I could manage more than an hour of focused attention at a time.

It is difficult to admit it but I found myself feeling resentful that Mum's mood had improved so much when I was away. It makes me feel I was responsible for her being so depressed and nasty.

But maybe I was. I was depressed and nasty myself before I went away. Had I not gone, I don't like to think what state I'd be in now. I also think it hugely unlikely that Mum's mood would have improved so much (if at all).

But now I am back.

My fear is that I am not going to be able to sustain this sense of relaxation for long, and that soon we'll be back where we left off.

Holidays are so important. But lots of carers don't take them. They convince themselves that only they can care for their piglet, or that their piglet will be traumatized by their absence. But if you don't have a holiday, your piglet might have to get used to more than your temporary absence. Do yourself (and your piglet) a favour. Book a holiday.

End of Tether One

It has all fallen apart. Despite my holiday, and Mum's being her cheerful self when I got back, ten days ago I reached the end of my tether.

The trigger was Carol's saying gently that she didn't think she could get Mum up any more.

I have been dreading this. But it had to come. Getting Mum up is truly *awful*. She hates to get up and, boy, does she let you know. It is difficult dressing her at the best of times because she no longer knows what goes where. It is often necessary, for example, to try to bend her arms for her so they will go into her cardigan, but you try bending someone else's arms – jolly difficult. Especially when they don't want their arms bent.

Mum sees no reason to help. In fact, she often wants positively to hinder. However patient you are she'll still kick you in the face as you try to put her socks on. Her look of malevolence and purpose as she does this is alarming in a Mum who used to be so kind and well-intentioned.

Looking after Mum has become a nightmare. A never-ending, 24-hour nightmare. Even the wonderful people at Willows, Mum's day care centre, are getting cautious. Her incontinence makes life very difficult for them. Not least because she is so aggressive when they try to change her.

Mum's delight in Andrej has mutated into impatience. So Anita cannot bring Andrej any longer. This means Anita can't come nearly as much as she used to. Setting up the care rota alone now takes two or three hours.

So when Carol dropped her bombshell I found my eyes filling with tears. Then I started to weep. I couldn't stop. The weeping became sobbing. This wouldn't stop either.

I didn't know what to do. I started to ring the doctor, then stopped, thinking, 'They'll take Mum away and put her in a home.' I rang a friend but her answering machine was on. Still I was sobbing.

Carol was devastated by my state, and felt terribly guilty. I tried to reassure her, but couldn't as I became more and more desperate. I knew I had to do something. But I didn't know what to do that wouldn't make it worse.

In the end I rang Ian and Betty, my lovely uncle and aunt. When they answered I could hardly say anything through my sobs. Ian reacted immediately: 'We'll be there in three hours,' he said.

He then rang my other uncle who lives nearer. When he and his wife, Dottie, arrived, an hour later, I was still sobbing. Then the emergency doctor arrived, made me swallow a tranquillizer, and rang Social Services.

No one answered.

My memory tells me that I hit the brick wall very suddenly. I thought I was managing until suddenly I wasn't. But re-reading the blog I can see that there was quite a build-up. Even holidays weren't helping: it was great to be away, but I came back to the same problems. Thank goodness that my family and Social Services were able to step in.

End of Tether Two

I have now been in my own home on my own for a whole week. I cannot tell you how wonderful it is. It is so *calm*. I had forgotten about calm.

I have been obsessively scrubbing, polishing, washing and tidying drawers. I have been hoeing, raking, weeding, mowing and staking. The whole place is beginning to look like a show-home.

I have decided I really like my house. It is not the house I would have chosen for myself. I bought it because it was so suitable for Mum. But over the years we have lived here I have made it my own. The garden, especially, gives me real pleasure.

The only things I am desperate to change completely – thanks to Fatcat and her peeing habits – are the carpets.

All this activity is hugely therapeutic. It is helping me to regain a sense of order and control. It is also keeping my mind off the places I don't want to go.

I don't, for example, want to think about Mum. She is with Ian and Betty down on the Kentish coast. Judy, my sister, is with them. Mum loves the sea. It triggers memories (emotional ones, at least) of her idyllic childhood in South Shields. I know she is safe and happy, and I don't want to think further than that.

I also don't want to think about the future. One thing is certain: I cannot look after Mum any longer. About this there is no doubt in my mind. I have cared for my parents for the last 13 years, for the last five on a 24-hour basis, and I have had enough. I cannot – will not – do any more.

Obviously I have had to do some thinking about the future. For a start, the crisis I described last week pushed the panic button at Social Services. Our care manager is desperately looking for somewhere for Mum to go until a place becomes available for her at the nursing home nearby where I'd 'like' her to go.

The funding people are also pulling out all the stops. It looks as if Mum might get 100 per cent NHS funding. If she doesn't we won't be able to afford the nursing home I like and we'll have to think again.

But even writing this is beginning to upset me. I can't *bear* the thought of Mum in a home. She will be confused and frightened. She will feel lost and alone. How can I *do* this to Mum?

But how can I not?

So I refuse to think about it, and concentrate instead on 'fussing' Fatcat. She is missing Mum something rotten.

The sense I had during this time of having just 'let go' was tangible. As every carer knows, the weight of responsibility lies very heavily on the shoulders of the main carer. Even if it isn't strictly true, we feel that everything depends on us and that we have to keep all the balls in the air. Letting go was petrifying, liberating and – by this point – necessary.

Optimism

Mum's whole personality is shot through with optimism. When Mum still did intellectual, it was also philosophically grounded: 'If you expect the best and it doesn't happen,' she would say, 'at least you've had the pleasure of anticipation.'

Mum's optimism sometimes manifested itself in denial. If, for example, an eagerly anticipated holiday didn't come up to scratch, Mum would talk it up. By the time she got home it had fulfilled every expectation.

The Alzheimer's has not diminished Mum's optimism. If anything, it has enhanced it. There was a time, when Mum was first diagnosed, that every book was 'the best book I've *ever* read', every meal 'the best meal I've *ever* eaten'. Mum's language became the language of superlatives, her interactions with others laced with compliments and appreciation. This continued, generally speaking, until she lost her language.

It's hardly surprising people warm to her, is it?

I have inherited Mum's optimism. Or perhaps I have learned it. Either way I expect the best, am disappointed if I don't get it, but bounce quickly back. I am also capable of denial.

This can be useful. It means that few situations are so bad that I can't see good in them, few so desperate that I can't convince myself that at least I have learned from them. If you are a carer you will see how such an attitude can help.

But it can also hinder. I am sure my unwillingness to accept how bad things were was a contributory cause to our recent emergency. It was important to me to convince myself that the situation hadn't really changed, at least not significantly, so no way was I going to tell anyone about the trouble I was really in. I didn't even acknowledge to *myself* the trouble I was really in.

All carers know that if they need help they must shout it from the rafters. A show of managing, especially a convincing one, is desperately counterproductive.

Others, after all, have a vested interest in taking a carer's appearance of being able to manage at face value. There isn't usually much they can do to help. Or, if there is, such help would involve them in more or less serious disruption.

If our care managers can convince themselves we're fine,

for example, their budget won't come under further threat. If our families can convince themselves we're fine, then they needn't consider doing more.

Maybe this is cynical. Perhaps it is only because carers are usually so good at managing that people seem so happy to assume they *are* managing. Even as everything disintegrates around them.

Optimistic carers, susceptible to denial, are a boon to the whole system.

Until they crack.

> Would a 'buddy' system help carers given to optimism and denial? If three carers met regularly (every fortnight?), all could be alert to changes that might lead to things getting out of hand for one of them. Three would mean no one would have to rely solely on their own instincts.

The Meaning of Life

Last night I went to a party in London. I just went. I didn't worry about what time I'd get back. I didn't book carers, nor did I make sure Mum's supper was prepared, her bed changed, or anything else at all.

I had a great time.

But twice I found myself saying: '... and I look after my Mum, who has advanced Alzheimer's'. Even as I uttered the words, I wondered why.

Of course I *am* still a carer – that Mum is currently with my brother and will soon go into a home doesn't mean I am not a carer. I am still responsible for liaising with Social Services, finances and, no doubt, visiting. (I *dread* the visiting.) It's too soon to think my caring days are over.

But I no longer have 'hands-on' responsibility. I don't brush Mum's teeth, change her pads, do her washing, deal with her moods … The really important part of being a carer is over.

So why am I still claiming to be a carer?

Perhaps I'm not yet out of the habit?

Habit? Is that the right word? I have cared for my parents for 13 years: my whole identity is shot through with being a carer. How can I stop thinking of myself as a carer just like that?

I didn't think of myself as a carer at all until Mum came to live with me. This is strange: caring from a distance can be worse than the hands-on stuff. I now know I was in that twilight world every carer goes through before they realize that there is help out there.

If the Government is to change carers' lot, it must get across to carers – and others – just who carers *are* and why they are important.

Yet the thing I hear most is that carers save the economy £87 billion a year.

Is this why carers are important? I don't think so.

Forget the economy. Carers are important because they look after those whom society would, I think, prefer to forget. Our society simply can't deal with the halt and the lame, the demented or the frail. We are far too busy securing bonuses to make a carer's eyes water, buying handbags at £500 a pop, building cars that go faster than any speed limit, and celebrating anyone who gets on TV.

Such activities may be fun but, compared to the activities of a carer, they are, in my opinion, utterly meaningless.

In making my lovely Mum's life meaningful, I was contributing to the meaning of my own life. To be a carer is, in my opinion, to be truly human.

No wonder I am reluctant to give up the title.

> The Carers' Centres count you as a carer even after your
> piglet has gone into a home. They continue to treat you as
> a carer, in fact, until one year after you stop caring. I think
> this is right. It took me ages to get used to Mum's being
> in a home. The caring, furthermore, doesn't stop. It just
> changes.

Poor Fatcat

Poor old Fatcat. She misses Mum terribly. She even stretches out
her paw to me. She must be desperate.

Every afternoon at around 3.30, when Mum used to come
home from day care, Fatcat asks to be let out. Once out she'll sit
alert and ready, looking at the road. You'd swear she was waiting
for the bus. She also butts me in the leg the way she used to butt
Mum. I try to fuss her, but not half as much as Mum did. It's not
surprising Fatcat misses her.

What's to be done about Fatcat?

The simplest thing would be to maintain the status quo. But
after reading this far, you'll know that Fatcat and I are not the best
of friends.

It's partly her peeing on the carpet. But now Mum has gone I
can shut a door and be sure it'll *stay* shut. This means I can keep
Fatcat out of the study and Mum's room during the day, and pen
her in at night so she can't get to her peeing spots. And she has
enough manners not to pee anywhere else.

But it's also that she's so fat she can't wash herself. So she sheds
her fur all over the place and, unlike Oedipus, she's not sleek and
shiny. She's sort of greasy. Yuk! Who wants to stroke a greasy cat?

I could put her on another diet now Mum's not here to
sabotage it. But could I bear to deny Fatcat her food? She has a
look I'm sure she reserves for me: a malevolent 'you can't get me'

look. I suppose it's reasonable after five years of my threatening to throw her out. But it doesn't endear her to me. It certainly doesn't encourage me to worry about her health.

One manifestation of Fatcat's missing Mum is that she has taken to chasing Oedipus. Regularly I now see Oedipus streak past with Fatcat in hot pursuit, tummy wobbling, at about half the speed. Perhaps her weight will sort itself out?

There is a charity, the Cinnamon Trust (see the Resources chapter, pages 275–84), devoted to caring for the pets of the elderly. I checked it out on the web. I am not sure it is suitable for Fatcat because it seems to require that the cat and its owner form a relationship with the Trust before there's a need. Nevertheless, I shall e-mail them.

I have, of course, considered taking Fatcat to the vet. But after all her years of devoted service to Mum, that strikes me as a betrayal too far.

I may not have been able to care for Mum until the end, but at least I can do it for her blasted cat.

> If you want to deter your piglet from entering or leaving a room (or going up or downstairs), make sure they'd have to step onto a black mat first. If they see it as a hole they'll be reluctant to go there. This worked for me.

A Waiting Game

I like to be doing things. I can't bear waiting. But at the moment waiting is the name of the game.

Funding is one thing we're waiting for. Mum apparently has a good chance of getting 100 per cent NHS funding. If she gets it, her only contribution to her own care will be the £130 a week she has been assessed as capable of affording from her state pension and her minuscule widow's pension. If she doesn't get 100 per cent funding she'll have to go into a cheaper home. Or the family will have to 'top up' her contribution, as we did with Dad.

Clearly the funding decision is an important one. I provided all the financial and other information months ago. No idea why it is taking so long.

But it's not as frustrating as it might be because we are also waiting for a bed. The home we're after, specializing in advanced dementia, has just had a new 20-bed wing built. You'd think that means 20 available beds, wouldn't you?

That shows how little you know.

The 20 beds cannot be allocated until they have been 'registered'. This, apparently, might take four months. FOUR MONTHS?? How can registering 20 desperately needed beds take four months? Are there hundreds of other new beds waiting to be registered? I doubt it. In the meantime, 20 carers – and their families – are at their wits' end.

When I last spoke to our care manager, Mum was classified as 'in crisis'. This puts her near the top of the list.

But Mum was in crisis because *I* was in crisis. Mum is now with my brother and his wife. I am no longer in crisis. Does this mean that Mum may be trumped by someone else? I wonder which crisis will result in Mum's actually getting into a home? How 'crisis-like' must a crisis be before something is done?

That there will soon be another crisis is obvious. My sister, who was travelling round the family with Mum, has had to go home suffering from stress. My brother and his wife, in their late sixties, are not in the best of health. My sister-in-law, in particular, has high blood pressure. Looking after Mum is not going to help that. My aunt and uncle, in their late seventies, managed ten days, in spite of my aunt's arthritis.

Although I am no longer the sobbing wreck of three weeks ago, I have reached the end of the road. Mum cannot come back to me. I wanted to see Mum through to her death. But I can't. End of story.

So Mum might not herself be in crisis, but those around her are dropping like flies.

Read the 'personal finance' pages of your newspaper. Subscribe to *Saga* magazine. Listen to 'Money Box' and 'You and Yours' on Radio 4. All are sources of useful information about benefits, changes to pension arrangements, care costs, looking after someone else's money and financial scams affecting the mentally vulnerable. Invaluable stuff, especially if you're unused to finance or if your financial situation is about to change.

Mercy Killing

We are still waiting. Every day I think of something else to worry about. What would happen, for example, if Mum were to be offered a place before we get the funding decision?

If we say 'yes' to the home but then the funding decision goes against us, we'll be in trouble. £900 per week is completely beyond us. Mum would have to be moved. Yet everything we're doing at the moment amounts to an attempt to avoid such a move.

But if we say 'no', then get the money, we'll have lost our place in the queue. No doubt we'd then have to wait months for another one.

It is **SO** frustrating!

I keep finding myself wishing Mum would die. If she were simply not to wake up one morning, it would be easier not just for her, but for everyone else.

During the last dreadful weeks I have often thought this. It is agonizing to hear the mother you love saying she's desperately unhappy. It is even more agonizing to be completely helpless in the face of such unhappiness. Whatever I said, Mum would have forgotten it ten seconds later and we'd go through the loop again.

If I had been sure I was doing it for Mum's sake I think I might have acted. In the last few months she has repeatedly said she wanted to die. But I'm not sure that *my* desire for her death wasn't stronger.

It would be one thing to end Mum's life for her own sake. It would be quite another thing to end it for MY sake. The first might be justified. The second could never be. There is, after all, an alternative – the alternative I am in fact taking.

Mum nursed her own mother through lung cancer in the days when there was little to be done for the pain. Mum often said she wished she'd had the courage to end her mum's suffering. I have been wondering if it is courage that is lacking in my case.

I don't think so. If I could be sure I wasn't acting selfishly I would be prepared to take the consequences. I certainly wouldn't try to hide my actions. It would be important to me that others should be free to make up their own minds about whether I had acted rightly or not.

I sense – and feel – the desperation of carers who have got to the point of no return on this decision. It is another decision that no one can make for anyone else. I am 100 per cent behind those who felt they had only one choice, and who were prepared to take the consequences.

But I am not, I think, in favour of legalizing mercy killing. Such legalization would, for a start, have to be so circumscribed that it would be useless for anyone in Mum's situation.

Mum has not been mentally competent for many years now: it would be ironic if the only decision she were deemed capable of making would be the decision to end her own life.

This blog was never published. The blog editor decided, I think, that it was too close to the bone. It also makes explicit my opinion on an extremely controversial issue. It is, though, such an important issue. How can a carer in the situation I was in *not* have an opinion on the issue? If you disagree, let's just agree this is an extremely difficult matter.

Sibling Rows

Aaargh!

ANOTHER assessment! So far, I'm told, we have had only the *preliminary* assessments. Well, of course.

At least we have a date. They're coming on Friday at 11 a.m. Poor Mum. She detests getting up early. But it will take two hours to get her back here. In this hot weather that won't be much fun. I suggested that the assessor and I travel to Mum. But no go. So much for the patient-centred approach.

But then another complication arose: when I rang my brother about the appointment, he dropped a bombshell. He and his wife and my sister have decided that Mum would be 'traumatized' by returning here. 'The assessment' he said 'will have to be somewhere else'.

I completely lost it.

They're telling me this NOW? Didn't they think of telling me *before* I finally succeeded in getting the appointment?

Anyway, what business have they 'deciding' this without me? How DARE they decide *anything* without consulting me?

The idea that coming here would traumatize Mum hurts. It implies that this house, where I loved and cared for her for so long, is a place of pain for Mum. But any pain Mum experienced here was integral to the Alzheimer's. Any other pain was mine. Even the final crisis was successfully kept from Mum. Mum just thought (if she thought at all) that she was going off with her brother for a holiday. She saw nothing of the tears, or the doctor's to-ing and fro-ing.

Perhaps my siblings think Mum would be traumatized by being reminded of, then removed from, her home? But if this is right it demonstrates their lack of a grip on Mum's condition.

For this to happen Mum would have to recognize this as her home, want to be here, recognize that she was only visiting and, putting all this together, become traumatized.

Dream on: Mum hasn't the foggiest idea where she is, never mind where she wants to be. I am only too aware of her emotional memory, but it isn't up to the sort of sophisticated reasoning this requires.

So I am furious with my siblings. And they think I am being unreasonable.

If you are a carer, this situation will be familiar. The carer slogs on until they hit a brick wall. Then everyone else weighs in with the wisdom that comes from knowing nothing. Then, when the carer goes ballistic, everyone shakes their head about how over-sensitive the carer is.

It is only at carers' get-togethers that you remember you are an ordinary human being doing a job that would drive even a saint mad. At that point it becomes funny.

But it doesn't feel in the slightest bit funny from where I am currently standing.

I suspect my siblings didn't consult me because they thought I was too traumatized myself. It is certainly true at that point that my decision-making skills were a little wonky. But so long as someone has been left in charge of the practical arrangements, I think they should be consulted on any decision affecting these arrangements. See Carers' Fury, pages 225–34.

The Assessment

The final assessment is over. The final *funding* assessment, anyway. We haven't even started with those to do with Mum's suitability for a home.

This one was awful. Not because of the assessment so much as the tension between me and my brother and sister-in-law. I continue to feel betrayed by their having decided, with my sister but without me, that Mum would be traumatized by returning to this house.

The atmosphere was full of my resentment, and everyone else's treading on eggshells.

I felt for the assessor, who had no idea what was going on. I hope she didn't think she was doing something wrong. Our care manager, who was sitting in, does know. She tells me such tension is completely normal when one sibling has done most of the caring.

As for trauma: Mum acted as if she had never seen the house before. She greeted me with affection, and maybe a spark of recognition, and asked politely where the lavatory was. She displayed none of the understanding on which trauma might be based (ha!).

She didn't even recognize Fatcat. I picked Fatcat up, hoping to stimulate Mum's old adoration. But Fatcat hates to be picked up and hissed violently. Mum recoiled, and later threw a handkerchief at poor old Fatcat.

The test started. The questions were amazing ... Mum wouldn't have been able to answer them three years ago, never mind now! Asked what year the First World War started she said, '1999'. Asked how old she was, she clearly had no idea. She was then given an address and told that in a few minutes she would be asked to repeat it.

Eh??

Mum has lived with me for nearly five years and hasn't been able to remember the address from day one. She had no idea even what she was being asked.

As the questioning proceeded ('What year are we in?' 'Who is Prime Minister?') Mum started to get upset. She still has a sense of when she is being tested. Once she loved to rise to the challenge, sometimes unhelpfully so, but now, I think she can sense only that she's failing.

Mum does not like to fail.

The rest of the assessment was directed at the carer. As I answered questions about Mum's mood and interaction with others, especially those caring for her, it came home to me again how utterly Mum has changed over the last six months.

I used to feel desperate at the thought of her going into a home. But as she is now I think a home is the only way she'll get the routine and security she needs.

I just hope she becomes institutionalized as soon as possible.

There's a whole radio station devoted to carers! Carers World Radio is devoted to providing information and advice to carers, a platform for carers to discuss their needs with policymakers, and they also want carers to participate in their programmes. There is also a chatroom. See the Resources chapter. I wish I'd known about this at the time I was writing this blog.

Nightmares

I had a dreadful dream last night. Mum and I were together. I knew, in the way you know in dreams, that we were at home, though it didn't look like it. I was trying to get Mum to rest. I was also trying to tidy up.

So much clutter! The faster I tried to tidy it, the more there was. I would put one lot away, check on Mum, then turn back to find it worse than before.

In the meantime, Mum was complaining loudly about being uncomfortable. She kept getting up and going into the next room. The next room was as cluttered as the first.

Mum started to iron. Suddenly the room was full of wet clothes. Mum was putting them to dry on the gas fires dotted around the place.

I became convinced the place was going to go up in flames. I tried to turn the fires down, but couldn't. Mum wouldn't stop loading them with damp clothes.

Then just as suddenly we were outside and Mum was haring off down the road with a couple who had appeared from nowhere.

I tore after them, but they went too fast. As I ran I was worrying about the possibility of fire. At the corner of the street I couldn't see Mum anywhere. It was tipping down with rain.

I woke with tears pouring down my cheeks.

Hmm.

My dreams have always worn their meanings on their sleeves. This one seems pretty obvious.

The attempts to clear up the clutter symbolize my desperate attempts, over the last six months, to keep up with everything I had to do. I was reduced in the end to comforting myself with lists – lists of all the things I should do, lists of all the things I *would* do if I could only find the time.

The fear of fire symbolizes my fear of dropping the balls. I am a person who likes to keep a lot of balls in the air. Occasionally I have dropped one. Over the last three months I have dropped so many, it is as if I have thrown down the rest.

The couple who came from nowhere are obviously my brother and sister-in-law. In my subconscious they have stolen Mum away from me.

This is not fair. Thank goodness they took Mum when they

did. However I might feel about them at the moment, I am absolutely confident they are looking after Mum as well as I did. In fact, given that there are two of them and they are retired, they are giving her the routine she needs and that I couldn't provide.

But my subconscious is obviously not a happy bunny.

> The whole family at this point was a bit of a mess. The focus of everyone's attention was Mum. But my needs were, I think, at least as important as Mum's. But not even I took them into account. Thank goodness for my friends. They suggested I seek counselling. Sadly I didn't. Perhaps you can learn from my mistake?

Running Away

When I was eight I ran away. I was wearing my blue chiffon party dress, mohair bolero and white shoes and socks. Worn only once, I wasn't about to leave them. I did leave a note blaming Richard (my brother) and saying no one should look for me.

After 20 minutes I found myself dying to go to the loo. Going behind a bush didn't appeal. So I knocked on a door and asked the nice lady if I could please use her lavatory.

Before I knew it I was in a police car going home. The policeman sternly told me he should be looking for burglars, not little girls. I was mortified.

It's in the genes. Dad regularly ran away from his nursing home. He once broke the window with the little fire hammer. Notwithstanding his dementia, and two busy roads, he would walk the three miles home.

Mum got used to looking up from whatever she was doing to see Daddy grinning through the window.

Dad's running away didn't help us get used to his being in a home. But it did tip him into the next funding classification. Every bit helps!

Some carers virtually become prison warders, so assiduously must they lock doors to keep their piglets from wandering. But Mum has only wandered three times.

The first episode seemed to me an entirely rational response to her treatment during that dreadful week of respite care. The second time she managed to get downstairs and into the front garden on a frosty night in January. Thankfully, neighbours saw her before she froze.

Then a couple of months ago, on a lovely sunny day, we were in the garden. I was sunbathing. Mum was complaining that she wanted to go home. I responded soothingly several dozen times, then snapped: 'Well, you know where the door is!'

I didn't actually think she *did* know where the door was. When she demonstrated that she did, I threw a pair of jeans over my swimming costume and followed her.

Clutching a red-and-white blanket over her blue sundress, a wide-brimmed white hat crammed on her head, she was walking determinedly down the road. She reminded me of Paddington Bear. I decided that, rather than stop her, I'd simply follow to make sure she didn't come to harm.

At the corner she hesitated, then turned right. At the next corner she hesitated again. Deciding enough was enough, I overtook her, greeted her with delight and asked if she was coming to see me. 'Yes' she said, unconvincingly. So I took her home and made a nice cup of tea.

I hope she's not going to be like Dad.

If your piglet is disabled and you have added a bathroom or kitchen to your house, or set aside a bedroom or sitting room for their use, or have had the house modified for a wheelchair, you might be eligible for a reduction in Council tax. Contact your local Council.

Moving Day

Today Mum moves into a nursing home.

It happened so suddenly. On Tuesday I was told that we were eligible for 100 per cent NHS funding. I was simultaneously warned not to feel too secure. If Mum becomes bed-ridden, and therefore easier to care for, she will lose this money. Oh, dear. Nothing like a bit of insecurity to keep you on your toes, is there?

Next I was told that we had a place in our chosen care home. It costs £900 per week. More than Eton!

I even got to choose Mum's room. This isn't normal, but the new extension has several rooms vacant. I chose a large, light, airy room at the end of a wide corridor. It has a pink carpet and pinky-grey curtains, large French windows opening onto a terrace, another window looking onto a grassy slope, and a huge sparklingly clean en-suite. It is delightful! I wouldn't mind moving in myself.

I'd have to change the loo seat, though. It is an alarming bright red.

The home has a music therapy room (Mum adores banging drums), a 'sensory room' with low music and coloured lights (good, I'm told, for when people are anxious), and gardens secure enough to allow people to wander. The residents seem happy. I saw one member of staff clasp a resident to her bosom and give her a smacking kiss!

It is even possible they'll take Fatcat. Now, that really *would* be something. I have said I'll pay for her keep and for a cat flap.

I spent yesterday sewing in name tapes, briefing the chef on coeliac disease and personalizing Mum's room. Mum's blanket is on her bed, the portraits of the four of us are on the wall opposite, her graduation photograph is next to the dressing table, and there are wedding and family photographs on her windowsill. I shall keep her supplied with flowers from the garden and soft fruit for her bowl.

I have been making a collage of photographs and writing a potted history for her door.

I feel very strange. I am pleased with the home, its delightful manager, and the fact we shan't (for the moment) have money worries. I have cheering fantasies about Mum's settling happily. I imagine her coming to tea with me, and taking her for walks around the gardens.

But I am warning myself that even if Mum does eventually settle, the transition period is likely to be painful. I hate the thought she might wake up alone and frightened, and I am haunted by visions of her traumatized face when she last spent time in a home.

But this time there is no alternative. Keep your fingers crossed for us …

> When your piglet goes into a home, don't even *think* of sewing on nametapes. I must have been mad. Get the iron-on ones, or an indelible marker pen that writes on fabric. Name *everything*: toothbrush, slippers, socks, handkerchiefs, bottles of shampoo and so on. Anything unnamed will disappear within minutes.

The First Week

Well, if you kept your fingers crossed for us, thank you! Mum has settled into her new home as if she were born to it. I am even losing my fear of visiting because I no longer expect her to be distressed. This is beyond my wildest dreams.

Last week I went in a special transport van to my brother's to collect Mum. On the way the driver Ray and I discussed how to tell Mum where we were taking her. I was sure Mum would constantly be asking 'Where are we going?' I didn't want to say 'home' because she might get excited, then disappointed (though goodness knows what she means when she asks to go 'home'). Nor did I want to say 'your new home' for fear of frightening her.

'Why don't you just say "Oxford"?' said Ray. Very sensible. Why didn't I think of that? But in the event Mum didn't ask once.

On arrival I was apprehensive. Unnecessarily so. Mum gave the manager, Elisa, who greeted us, a bear hug and a smacking kiss. She did the same to the first carer we met.

As we walked in procession towards Mum's room, I said nervously: 'We're going to see your new room. You'll love it.'

'That's nice' said Mum, vaguely. She was more interested in a woman we were passing who seemed to be crying. 'Oh, dear' said Mum, putting her arms around her, 'it'll be all right, you'll see.' Everyone looked at me with one of those 'aaah!' expressions. I felt inordinately proud. The woman grabbed Mum's hand and joined our procession.

Mum thought her room was lovely. I kept repeating that it was her new room, expecting her to realize what was going on and protest. But no, she accepted it without question.

The carer took her to have a cup of tea whilst I unpacked. I re-joined them, again apprehensively. But Mum was engrossed in animated and unintelligible conversation with another resident. Good old Mum – her social instinct is still alive.

So I said I was going. And I went.

I had a bad night imagining her sleepless in a strange bed. But when I rang the next morning I heard that she had been fine, despite having been up until 6 a.m.

Every day I have visited her. Every day she has been fine. Yesterday I found her tormenting a carer with a rubbery orange toy. The carer was enjoying being teased, and Mum was in fine fettle.

I have heard about people unexpectedly taking to nursing homes. I couldn't believe we'd be that lucky. Perhaps Mum's gaddings about over the last few weeks smoothed the way?

But whatever the explanation I am everlastingly grateful. Perhaps I am about to get my life back?!

> Write a short biography of your piglet. Include special interests and hobbies. Illustrate it with photographs of them in their prime – the beautiful bride, the thrusting executive, the proud gardener – then laminate a copy for each substitute carer and/or for the door of their room in the nursing home. Talk to all the staff about what your piglet was like when younger.

Birthday

It was Mum's 89th birthday on Saturday. When I visited, there was a party in progress. There were 'Happy Birthday' banners on the wall and the door, and Mum was in her favourite chiffon outfit. Very Queen Mum! Though I doubt Her Majesty ever had fingernails of that particular violent pink.

There were two cakes: a chocolate gluten-free one just for Mum, another for everyone else. Mum was singing away, surrounded by a respectable number of birthday cards, all featuring cats.

I stayed half an hour. Ideal. The whole thing is ideal and I am feeling incredibly happy. The home is 10 minutes' cycle ride away, so it is easy to take half an hour out and spend 10 minutes with Mum. It is also on my route to and from town so I can drop in after my swim, or before a meeting.

Mum doesn't seem to mind that I only stay 10 minutes. It is a really enjoyable 10 minutes. I fetch her glasses and we 'read' together. Then I say 'I'm off! See you tomorrow' and she puts up her face for a kiss.

All this is enabling me to re-engage with my love for her. During the last dreadful six to nine months it has been so difficult to access this love. How can you love someone who is querulous, demanding and difficult? Try as I did, I found myself disliking her more and more. But now loving her is as easy as it ever was.

Looking back, Mum should have gone into a home about six months ago. Re-reading my blog I see there was a point at which I was thinking she was no longer getting any benefit from being looked after by me, that what she really needed were professionals. But I was arrogant enough to believe that no one could look after her as well as I could, frightened by our dreadful experience of respite, and frankly I was just too exhausted to be able to see straight.

As the situation became more and more intolerable I patched and patched it, adding this and dropping that until I hardly even knew what I was doing.

But of course it wasn't just my failings that led to the delay. The whole system is set up in such a way that people in Mum's position rarely get what they need until they, and of course, the person caring for them, are literally unable to cope. In order for the system to grind into action I had to get myself into such a state I was prescribed valium (I can heartily recommend it). Mum was put through six months of agony and so was I.

There must surely be a better way?

> When your piglet goes into a home, if there are clothes that matter to you – that expensive linen jacket, the jumper you or your piglet hand-knitted, the tie your grandchildren saved for – keep them at home. The nursing home hasn't time for such niceties. They'll all end up in the same wash. The boil-wash.

Alarming Phone Calls

Yesterday the home rang to say Mum had fallen over. They found her on the floor. No harm done. After a hot drink she was fine.

But it brought home the fact that one day I might get a more serious call.

That's what happened with Dad. Four of my friends were due for supper. Everything was ready, table laid, wine opened, then the phone rang. It was Richard. Dad had been taken into hospital after a choking fit. I should come straight away.

There is nothing worse than being 200 miles away and carless at such a time.

I rang rail enquiries, and amazingly there was a train in 45 minutes. Just time to fling a bag together and hare off to the station. One of my friends arrived as I was unchaining the bike. I left her, rather bewilderedly, in charge of a supper party, which apparently went well, though dampened by the reason for my disappearance.

On the train I tried to collect my thoughts. But they wouldn't be collected. They skittered and slid from one irrelevance to another. Some things are too big to think about.

An hour into the journey my phone rang: Dad had died.

For some reason that doesn't make any sense now I think about it, I was given the news by a friend rather than by one of my family. This particular friend had lost his own father when he was six. He was almost more distressed to give the news than I was to receive it.

The rest of the journey is something of a blur. I remember the conductor, face a picture of sympathy, coming to say that my sister had rung to say they'd be waiting at the station (maybe they didn't have my phone number?). Then, clearly desperate to help, he brought me tea and a muffin. I felt I had to eat it. It was like sawdust.

Richard and Judy were at the station. On the way to the hospital I became panicky thinking I might be confronted with Dad's body before I was ready. It wasn't a problem of course. I sat at the nurse's station (yet more tea) until I was ready. Then I went in.

Funnily enough, it was OK.

Poor Dad. All the juice had gone from him. He was so thin, so racked by emphysema, that his death was a blessing. Even Mum couldn't find it in her heart to want to call him back.

The week of the funeral was strange. So much, and yet nothing, to do. The funeral itself was comforting: the church was full and I felt we had done Dad justice. He was a good man.

> It was after this phone call that I thought to take Mum's Living Will to the home so they knew her wishes should there be a 'life-threatening incident'. I was very glad I did because I should never have thought of it when that life-threatening incident did occur. See pages 249–60.

Speedfreak

I spent last week in the New Forest. I go every year, always to the same place. Such a creature of habit. For the past five years I have taken Mum. Mum loved the view over the lawns to the Solent. She exclaimed whenever ferries passed (often), especially at night with all their lights twinkling, and she loved to see the masts of the sailing boats swaying. She also loved to see the ducks come right onto the terrace for bread.

But I have to say that, this time, what *I* loved was not having Mum with me.

Such pleasure to go walking when I wanted, for as long as I wanted. So good to have people over for lunch and supper, and to be as noisy as I liked without fear of disturbing her. Bliss.

But even more blissful, in fact completely, utterly *wonderful*, was getting home and finding the house empty and exactly as I'd left it!

For nearly five years every time I've come home it has been to a house full of people, an upside-down kitchen, and nothing where I would expect it. Instead of being able to unpack and lower myself back into everyday life, I'd find myself socializing with whoever was caring for Mum. Then, when they left, having to take over the caring.

I'd find myself unpacking at midnight, as I parried Mum's nocturnal forays, and then before getting Mum up for day care and going to work, I'd have to face all the e-mails, mail and telephone calls that had piled up whilst I was away. Within 24 hours I'd feel as stressed as I did before I went away.

This time I opened the front door and drank in the silence. I wandered from room to room loving the fact that everything was where it should be. I unpacked my case into the washing machine, opened my mail, dealt with phone messages and e-mail, and within a couple of hours I was able to relax with a glass of wine. It was completely magical.

On my way home from the station I called in on Mum. She recognized me immediately and was touchingly pleased to see me. It was sunny and warm so I suggested I take her in her wheelchair round the gardens. I warned her she'd have to behave or I'd spin her chair round. When I demonstrated, she egged me on to do just that. Then instead of walking her round, I *ran* her round, talking about when she and Daddy used to do 'the ton' on his motorbike. Mum was giggling delightedly and insisting I go faster and faster.

She was always a speedfreak.

Your piglet might have lost their cognitive skills, their memory and even their language and yet still be physically fit, healthy and enthusiastic. If this is the case you'll both benefit from lengthy walks, games like 'catch', football and 'tag'. They'll enjoy it and may sleep better. And so might you.

Conferences

Yesterday Mum was a star at the Conservative Party Conference. Carers UK had asked me to participate on their behalf in a debate with Stephen O'Brien MP and Tim Hammond, the MD of Barchester Homes. It was chaired by Martyn Lewis (yes, the one you used to see on television every night). It was great fun. I hope no one could see my hands shaking.

Just before the debate Terry Pratchett, the author, spoke. He has just been diagnosed with Alzheimer's and is using the energy occasioned by this to campaign on behalf of those with the disease. He has donated £½ million to Alzheimer's research. I was uncomfortably aware of him as I spoke. I didn't pull punches about Mum's condition: how dreadful to have to listen – in public – to a graphic account of the nightmare to come. A brave man (and fun too, as I discovered over drinks afterwards!)

I started by showing a slide of Mum aged 17, the one in which she looks like Catherine Zeta-Jones. I think it is important to remind people that she was once young, vital and full of dreams. Then I showed them a picture of Mum now. As I spoke they could see both pictures.

First I told them about Mum's condition, describing everything from her joyous sense of fun and her love of children, to her weeping and desperate desire to die. I talked of her incontinence, her need to be fed and her inability, now, even to dress herself or construct a meaningful sentence. Finally I talked about being Mum's carer; the sleepless nights, the despair, the guilt, the tears and the pain as well as the love, laughter and joy. I'd like to think there wasn't a dry eye in the house.

Afterwards lots of people came to talk to me. Everyone spoke of their mum/dad/aunt/granny. So many people, so many personal tragedies.

But so telling. The fact is that the end of life, with all its woes, is part of life. Few of us will escape untouched by the need to care or be cared for at the end. Sometimes, sadly, as with Terry, before the end.

Yet as every carer knows to become a carer is to become invisible.

Invisible, helpless and, all too often, hopeless. How can this be? How can even the most minor 'celebrity' command more column inches in our newspapers than this army of people who – unpaid and unlauded – are doing one of the most important jobs a person can do?

I hope the fact that at least one of the main political parties is addressing the issue is a sign this might change.

But I don't think I'll hold my breath.

> Put yourself onto the media lists of organizations such as Carers UK, the Alzheimer's Society, the Princess Royal Trust for Carers and so on. Then, when they have a story that needs a quote from, or pictures of, carers they can call on you. It makes the story stronger and helps to alert the rest of the world to our existence.

Soaring Spirits

To my astonishment I am really enjoying my visits to Mum. She has returned to being so wonderfully herself. When I think back to four months ago ... it is a whole new world!

It is interesting to speculate on this extraordinary change.

Is it that she has regained her freedom? When she was with me she was never allowed to just get up and go: someone would always be following her, asking her where she was going and offering to get for her whatever it was she wanted.

Now I think about it, it must have been irritating beyond belief.

But now she can go anywhere she likes. She can walk the long, wide corridors and stare through the big picture windows into the courtyards. She can even go into the gardens if she likes because, during the day, the doors are never locked. The perimeter fence is secure and obscured by prickly bushes, so the residents can't actually get out of the grounds. But within the grounds they can go wherever they like, when they like.

'Yes', said the director, when I asked, 'they might fall over. But we think it is better to take that risk and give them their freedom than that we are always restricting them.' Well, I couldn't agree more, if this is helping Mum be so cheerful.

Or perhaps Mum was unhappy because she was always being dragged from pillar to post? I had to work. So she had to go to day care. This meant she had to be prised from her bed far earlier than suited her, washed, dressed, breakfasted and pushed through the door the minute the bus came. Then she was driven around for two hours collecting other people, then she spent a few hours at the day centre before going through the whole process again in reverse. It makes me tired just thinking about it.

Now she can live life as it suits her, she can get up when she wants, go to bed when she wants and do what she wants.

Finally, I suspect it must be a relief no longer to be constantly the focus of attention. With me she was usually with just one carer at a time. This meant that she was always supposed to be *doing* something, talking or drawing or whatever. Now she can just sit. And just sitting doesn't mean that there isn't anything to entertain her. In the home there is always so much going on that it is easy to occupy yourself without actually having to do anything; you can just watch the world go by. What a relief this must be.

But whatever the explanation Mum's spirits are soaring, and so are mine!

In reading this I remember how terrified I was about Mum's going into a home, and how absolutely wonderful it was – for her and for me – when she did. If you too are petrified about your piglet's going into a home, be aware this might happen for you, too. I shall keep my fingers crossed for you.

Maive

I spent the weekend with my nephew, his wife and their two children. It was Anna's fifth birthday on Saturday and she had a party. I enjoyed myself enormously. I can't remember when I last played pass the parcel. (When did they start wrapping presents in each layer?)

Mum used to adore Anna and her brother Jacob, who will soon be seven. This adoration was mutual. Now Mum is settled in her home I have invited the children and their parents to stay so we can all visit Mum. It would be lovely if, when they're grown, they have some memory of her, and of the fun they had with her.

When I got home there was an ominous message on my answering machine. It was from the son of the second of Mum's best friends. I have never met this son, and there could only be one reason he'd be ringing me ...

... and so it proved. Maive died suddenly last Wednesday.

Funnily enough it was the same thing that killed Mum's other best friend, Pam: a burst aorta. Pam died in the middle of a game of bridge, as she was telling an anecdote about her time in the Wrens. Maive died as she was changing for bed after a night out with friends.

Way to go, eh? Shocking for the family, but wouldn't you choose that if you could?

I am so sorry about Maive. She was a complete star. Spending time with Maive couldn't but leave you with a smile on your face. I never knew her to be anything but optimistic, and her laugh was infectious. Being groomed mattered very much to her: her nails were always perfect, as was her make-up.

I always think of Maive, Mum and Pam as being as thick as thieves. But this can't have been the case: Maive and Pam came from different parts of Mum's life.

Maive and Mum met, just after the war, when both had young children and lived in the same block of flats. They seemed to live for the time when, husbands gone to work, they could hang a duster in the window to signal the coast was clear, and spend the day in irreverent laughter.

Pam and Mum met much later, though again when both had young children (both had two 'sets' of children). But the laughter was the same.

Mum had, indeed has, a gift for friendship. When she got Alzheimer's and started to deteriorate, I got to know her friends on my own account. To a woman they are, or were, an admirable bunch.

As one by one they die, or succumb to dementia, I hope that we, the next generation, are worthy of them.

I thought it important that Mum should have the news about Maive. I didn't for one minute think she'd understand. Amazingly, I think she did. She looked sombre, then said, quite clearly 'Thank you for telling me.' I was very glad I had told her.

The Comfort of the Physical

Unforgivably, Mum gave my sister and me Dad's legs. How I longed for her legs. Long, slim, shapely. Racehorse legs.

I loved it when, family together for the evening, Dad would exclaim: 'You have very nice legs, dear!' bringing Mum's newspaper down in a flurry of giggles and blushes. Occasionally I'd come across them kissing. Cue embarrassed jumping apart, more giggles, more blushes.

Perhaps unusually for a 1950s childhood, I never learned that sex wasn't nice. It was clearly the rock on which my parents' marriage was built. Far from perfect, their relationship at least never lacked intimacy.

Dad's stroke did not destroy his sex drive. His understanding of *when* sexual behaviour was appropriate, sadly, *did* disappear.

Dad's lack of sexual inhibition was not directed at other women. Seeing Mum, however, he would immediately grab at her. This was distressing for her. Not least, I think, because she too missed their intimacy. Dementia and double incontinence don't half diminish your suitability as a sexual partner.

What an excruciating combination of guilt and loneliness must be triggered by finding yourself suddenly repulsed by your lifetime partner.

In his nursing home Dad acquired a new 'wife'. Louise used to sit next to him, holding his hand, chattering away at him and telling everyone he was her husband. This did not go down well with Mum. It is to her credit that she never did more than pierce Louise with gimlet eyes and put a dangerous tone into her '*I* am his wife.'

But I don't think Mum really felt threatened. Dad was so obviously a one-woman man. His 'relationship' with Louise was visibly one-sided. It was on seeing Mum that his eyes would light up.

But the fact remains: Dad's stroke brought a sudden end to a fulfilling and active sexual partnership. Mum went overnight from being a woman whose attractions were actively acknowledged by her husband, to someone whose sexuality was an embarrassment.

This is why I adore men who are prepared to flirt with, and robustly hug, Mum and other elderly women. My pal Ian, for example, always greets Mum with a huge sustained bear hug, and a compliment on her beauty. Mum visibly grows three inches. Her delight is a thing of wonder.

Peter, one of her carers, is another such man. He dances with her, holding her tight and twirling her. She gets quite pink. For just a moment Mum is not an elderly lady in a nursing home, but a beautiful woman tripping the light fantastic in the arms of an attentive man. It makes me smile just to think of it.

> Does your piglet go in for inappropriate sexual behaviour? Many do. Mum used to flirt outrageously with tall men. I found it cringe-making. I didn't find any way to stop it. But I did notice that the men rarely worried about it. Indeed, most gently flirted back. Feign an air of everything being perfectly normal.

Carpe Diem

None of the residents of Mum's home is hot on memory. But they're beginning to recognize me, and I am learning their names and habits.

There's one lady, Jane [all residents' names have been changed], who likes to hold hands. You'll be standing talking and suddenly you find your hand in an iron grip. Once she's got you there's no escape until you can get a carer to slip her hand between yours and Jane's so they can be prised apart.

Then there's the cheerful Tom, who loves to flirt. He's great fun. Mum loves to flirt, too, so I have been trying to put them together. They flirt nicely for 20 seconds, then lose interest. It's a shame; I'm sure it would enhance both their lives to spend them flirting with each other.

Then there's Sally with the wide smile, who spends her time marching up and down the corridors, and Ruth who does the same.

Last time I visited Mum I saw Ruth go up to another resident, an elderly lady asleep in her chair, smack her and take her blanket. The poor old dear was startled awake, clutching her ear in panic. I shopped Ruth to the carers. They remonstrated. But I could see Ruth didn't understand a word.

Some of the residents are much less advanced in their dementia than Mum. They can almost hold a proper conversation. I wonder how they feel about being in the home? Others are distressingly young. One is in his late forties. Life really isn't fair, is it?

I often visit Mum just as supper is being served so I can encourage her to eat. She really needs the encouragement: weight continues to fall off her and she is now painfully thin. Almost impossible to remember the lusty appetite she used to have.

The trouble with this regime is that I shall get fat. The best way to encourage Mum to eat is to eat with her. But I never eat quite enough with Mum to feel I've had supper. So at home I eat again. This must stop.

Visiting can be amazingly humbling. At the home everything goes at snail's pace. There's no point in rushing: no one can move fast, no one can understand if you speak quickly, and it can take an hour to finish a meal. One has time, and plenty of opportunity, to reflect on the human condition.

Visiting Mum doesn't half focus my mind on the fact that life is for living *now* rather than later. It's easy to forget this during daily life when everyone is rushing and there's never enough time.

But not if every night you get a vivid reminder of the way you might end up.

If your piglet is in a nursing home and capable, to some degree, of feeding themselves, you might want to go in at mealtimes for a while to check they are eating enough. The carers will be busy with those who need feeding. They might – wrongly – think your piglet left all their food because they weren't hungry.

Gluten Enthusiasm

I am worried about Mum's diet. I think the home – with the best will in the world – may be being a little overenthusiastic with her gluten-free diet.

When Mum moved in I went to meet the chef so I could be sure he understood Mum's diet. It was very pleasing: I left with the impression he saw it as an interesting challenge.

The other staff were all told that Mum has coeliac disease, and given graphic descriptions of what happens when her diet is broken.

But I think there may still be some misconceptions.

Last week, for example, I visited Mum at lunchtime. They were serving battered fish, chips and peas, and rice pudding. But Mum was struggling with a solid-looking gluten-free pizza served with boiled potatoes. For pudding she had a plateful of melon and pear pieces.

The batter on the fish made it a definite no-no. But Mum could easily have had fish in some sort of cornflour-thickened sauce. This would have been much easier for her. Poor old Mum only has one tooth at the front, and eating the pizza was obviously too daunting, especially as it became cold and the cheese congealed.

I tried cutting it into small bits. I tried eating some myself ('uuummm, delicious!'). I tried feeding her the scraped-off topping. But it was all too much. Mum just isn't a member of the pizza-eating generation.

As for the boiled potatoes – well, why? No reason why Mum couldn't have had chips. Mum *adores* chips.

Mum also likes melon and pear (she used to describe herself as a 'fruit bat'). But every time I have been with her at a meal time recently she has had melon and pear. It must be getting a bit boring.

Anyway, just between us, Mum and I would occasionally treat ourselves by eating whole tins of rice pudding. We LOVE rice pudding (especially tinned rice pudding). It is possible that the home uses a gluten-rich rice pudding. But gluten would be an unusual ingredient in rice pudding. I suspect they were just being cautious.

Obviously I'd rather they were cautious than reckless. But it is important that Mum be given food that is appetizing and easily manageable: she is so thin she can't afford to lose more weight.

The home is, I think, relying too heavily on ready-made stuff. But some of this stuff is inedible. The bread Mum gets on prescription, for example, has to be toasted or even the birds won't eat it. Ready-made biscuits are slightly better, but only slightly.

It makes me want to cry when Mum gets two anaemic-looking gluten-free chocolate 'bourbons' whilst others get freshly-baked scones with jam and cream.

The lacy napkins you use for guests? Forget them. For your piglet it isn't a napkin you need but an apron. And – once your piglet is past worrying about such things – one of those plastic bibs children use. A sheet of plastic under your piglet's chair isn't a bad idea, either. This is what they do in nursing homes.

Social Skills

When Mum lived with me I was often asked how I felt about her decline. I never knew how to answer because to me it was not her decline that mattered but her cheerfulness.

Mum is the most optimistic, cheerful, open and loving person I know. Unless she is in pain, being with her enhances life no end (so long as you 'stay in the moment').

I thought about this recently when I read about some new research that suggests our fear of dementia is misplaced. Many people who actually *have* dementia do not, apparently, experience any decline in their sense of wellbeing.

If you are lucky enough to be a happy person, in other words, getting dementia won't make you unhappy.

But, continues the research, this depends on your maintaining your social life: to become socially isolated is to invite anxiety and depression.

This chimes completely with my experience. Before Mum came to me, she was becoming isolated. She felt too vulnerable to go out and spent a huge amount of time alone. She started to get depressed.

She perked up when she came to live with me. But as she became more dependent I couldn't provide the social interaction she needed. So she started going to a day care centre. What a difference! Mum became herself again – outgoing and cheerful, loving and feisty. The lovely staff at the centre had the time, the patience and the expertise to interact with Mum and with the others as *people*. They listened to them, talked to them and made them feel valued. It gave Mum a new lease of life.

I think it is very easy for carers to think they know exactly what their piglets need. I was convinced Mum would hate day care. In retrospect I was imposing on Mum my own feelings, the feelings of someone *without* dementia.

Having seen Mum coming into her own again by going to day care I am convinced the research is right: maintain your social skills by going to somewhere like Willows and dementia needn't be the end of your enjoyment in life.

I have seen the same phenomenon in Mum's move to her nursing home. Once again Mum has been saved from the threat of social isolation. Although 20 years ago she would have *detested* the thought she'd end up somewhere like this, as she is now, it is just what she needs and she is thriving.

So having dementia can be consistent with living an enjoyable life. What a strange thought.

Now all we need is some way of enabling *carers* to maintain their social interactions so they too can avoid anxiety and depression!

> It is important, I think, to recognize that the things your piglet would have hated 20 years ago, are now, to your piglet, a matter of no moment. If you keep harking back to them as they used to be, it will be difficult to see that they might actually – as they are now – be quite enjoying life.

Driving

When I was 17 I wanted, like everyone else, driving lessons. This desire waned significantly when Dad came over all portentous: 'I'll teach you to drive,' he said, 'as soon as you demonstrate you know how an engine works'.

This is not what a 17-year-old girl wants to hear.

It got worse when Dad decided to instruct me himself. He was never going to be content with my knowing where to put the anti-freeze and how to check the oil. He was an engineer. He loved engines. He was going for the full monty.

Mum was more amenable. 'Huh,' she snorted, on hearing what Dad had said, 'Perhaps I should tell him he can eat supper when he demonstrates he knows how to cook it?'

So Mum took me out in her car. It wasn't a success. Driving back from church one Sunday, I took a corner too quickly and nearly hit another car. Mum made me stop, smoked a whole cigarette, and insisted we swap places. She never took me out again.

Since then I have lived only in places where cars are a liability, and I have never had children. I have managed to get to 53, therefore, without learning to drive.

But suddenly things are different. After five years of caring for Mum, and now that she has gone into a home, I am free to do anything I want. What I want is something that will stop me thinking of myself as a carer. I want out of the comfort zone I have built up over five years of responsibility.

So a friend and I did a brainstorm. I suggested taking a house in Croatia for a year. It would have a swimming pool and be big enough for friends to stay. My work I can do anywhere, and I should so love to spend a year in the sun.

Then Joanna, who thought this a wonderful idea, suggested we drive there. 'But,' she added, 'you would have to drive, too, I'm not doing it all by myself.'

The seed was planted. The following week it took root. Why not? I thought. So I booked a series of lessons.

Yesterday I had my ninth two-hour session. My instructor had me driving around the ring road at 60 mph. My heart was beating very fast. (It's possible his was beating faster.) I didn't like doing 60, but afterwards 30 seemed too slow. Perhaps I'm going to be a girl racer?

The important thing, though, is that I am loving it. And there's no doubt that, as I hang on to the steering wheel for dear life, I am not thinking of anything to do with caring.

> Enjoy the convenience of a car without bothering to own one. My local car-share scheme will rent you a car for an hour (or more) at a time. It is £4 per hour, and 15p per mile for petrol. There's also a one-off joining fee and a returnable charge for insurance.

Communication

Visiting Mum, I always glance at the noticeboard. The notices about music therapy, visiting chiropodists and outings keep me up with Mum's world.

Yesterday there was a different sort of notice: it announced the death of a resident. Not recognizing her surname, I checked. It was the lady I had in mind.

This means that her husband, a sad-faced man in his mid-eighties, will be grieving. I'd often seen him holding her hand. There wasn't much else he could do because she communicated only in a strange rhythmic grunt. Perhaps this wasn't even a communication but a tic.

But it was her eyes that always struck me. They had a look of quiet desperation. It was as if she wanted something, but knew she could do nothing about it.

Sometimes Mum's eyes have the same look. I hate it. It makes me feel helpless.

Writing that made me feel selfish. It should be Mum's quiet desperation I worry about, not my own feeling of helplessness. But there is no point in worrying about Mum's quiet desperation, if indeed that's what it is: there is nothing I can do about it.

Once I have checked she is comfortable, not in pain, hungry or thirsty, there's little else I can do. Thinking she might be bored, I try to read or sing with her, but she'll have none of it. Nor does she want to go for a walk or ride in her wheelchair.

I imagine the parents of a child who constantly cries feel the same. Loving someone who cannot tell you what they want is extremely frustrating.

Mum can speak. But she can't communicate. Her utterances are mostly unintelligible. I suppose they *have* meaning, because she seems to speak intentionally. I can see, for example, when she is asking a question. It might even be possible to guess what the question is about. But no way is it possible to guess what the question *is*.

Sometimes this doesn't matter. Mum is obviously just chatting. All I have to do is I respond arbitrarily, matching my tone to hers. 'When will the cup reach forever?' she asks. 'Oh, not for ages yet.' I reply. 'Good,' says Mum.

A conversational triumph!

Other times Mum obviously wants to communicate, but can't. Sometimes this frustrates her. Other times she seems sadly resigned.

Could a Fairy Godmother reveal Mum's thoughts? This assumes Mum has thoughts to reveal. Does she? Or are her thoughts as scrambled as her expression of them? I don't suppose I'll ever know.

Yesterday, however, we sang about 20 repeats of 'What shall we do with the drunken sailor?' (first verse only because I couldn't remember the rest). Mum seemed fine.

> I think being a bit of a performer helps no end when visiting a nursing home. Entering into their world is definitely the best way to communicate, and to make your visit feel productive. I rather enjoy talking friendly and cheerful nonsense for half an hour.

Where Is She?

Quite a to-do a couple of days ago. Went to visit Mum but she was nowhere to be found. I looked in all the sitting rooms and in the music room. She wasn't in the conservatory, nor in her own room. I checked the loos, the bathrooms and even the linen cupboards. No Mum.

I wasn't worried because, without in the least bit seeming to be, the home is very secure. But there was nothing left to do but recruit some of the staff to search the rooms of other residents.

We soon found her. She was fast asleep, tucked up in the bed of one of the other residents. It is possible she had been feeling ill. Certainly she had been – er – unwell. She badly needed changing, the bed badly needed new sheets (at least), and the room badly needed a scrub. Poor Mum.

The staff were, as always, wonderful. I just left them to it. It is one of the nicest things about Mum's being in a home that I can do this. When Mum lived at home I was constantly having to change her, wash her clothes and sheets, scrub carpets, etc. My washing machine thinks it's been made redundant.

None of the rooms in the home is locked. This means that residents can go in and out of each others' rooms at any time. One day I found Ruth in Mum's room, naked to the waist, in the process of shredding the water-resistant material of her knickers. It looked as if it had been snowing.

I just greeted her warmly, shut the door firmly, and went to find a member of staff.

Another time Tom was in Mum's room searching for something. He was obviously failing, because every drawer in the room was open, its contents strewn over the floor. He had reached the wardrobe when I got there, and was discarding garments one by one in disgust.

'Hi, Tom,' I said. 'I'll get someone to help you.' And off I went.

After five years of being responsible for everything, this ability to walk away is magical.

When Mum went into the home I was told to put her name on everything. I thought I had done so. But I interpreted 'everything' rather narrowly. They really mean that her name must be on every sock, her glasses, every book, every photograph, etc. If it isn't, whatever it is will go walking.

Actually it goes walking anyway. Mum's drawers are full of stuff that isn't hers, and I am sure that much of her stuff is being put to good use elsewhere.

But who cares? Mum certainly doesn't. So long as Mum is happy, neither do I.

When your piglet goes into a home, resolve to accept that you will often see them dressed in a strange assortment of other people's clothes. It isn't (always) the home's fault. If your piglet has an accident, the priority is (rightly) to get them into something clean, dry and warm as quickly as possible.

Mum as She Was Before

I passed the theory and hazard-perception part of my driving test last Thursday! I was ridiculously pleased. Friends congratulated me, but most added: 'O*f course* you did.'

I can see why they think this. But, for me, learning to drive is a *huge* step outside my comfort zone. I wanted champagne and cries of delight.

Thinking about this, a hollow opened in my tummy. I realized that the person I really wanted to tell was Mum. I had to fight back tears.

Incredibly, it is years since I have had an impulse based on thinking of Mum as she used to be before the Alzheimer's. I think this is extremely promising.

It is perhaps a sign that, after all the years of caring for Mum, the time is coming when I might again be able to think of her as my Mum, instead of as my responsibility.

That sounds bad. I do not mean that during the years of caring for her I haven't thought of her as my Mum. It is rather that the Mum she has been over the last 12 years is not the Mum she was before. It was to the Mum she was before that I wanted to talk to about my test success.

That Mum would have whooped with pleasure. She would have made me feel that my pleasure was hers. My pleasure *would* have been hers. Her generosity in such things was wonderful.

I used to think all mums were like this. But then, at a wedding once, I said to the bride's mum, 'She looks wonderful, you must be so happy.' Her mum replied grumpily, 'I'm glad you think so, but it's about time, isn't it?' I was shocked to the core. It wasn't so much the suggestion the bride had been almost on the shelf (she was 29!) as her mum's meanness of spirit. How does one's self-esteem survive such a mum?

Perhaps this is unfair? Perhaps her mum was having a bad day? But the incident has stayed in my mind, attached to heartfelt thanks that my mum was so different.

Mum wasn't blinkered in her belief in me. On the contrary, she was the first to say if she thought I was wrong, or that I had acted badly. But I never felt she was getting at me, and I never questioned her total support.

It will be wonderful to remember, and mourn, Mum as she used to be. Until now I have been too busy fire-fighting to do anything but take Mum as she comes. My impulse to tell her about my test suggests Mum's having gone into a home may mark the beginning of this process.

I do hope so.

I still think of Mum far more often as she was in her final years than as she was before. In dreams, for example, she is still very much the person I had to look after rather than the person she used to be. But I notice that as time passes this is changing. I am confident that, over time, my memories will be of her as she was when she was in her prime.

South Africa

For years after Dad had his stroke I had planned to take Mum to South Africa. My fear of flying always got in the way. Then I was told about Mum's Alzheimer's. The diagnosis trumped my fear and the holiday was booked.

Mum's dad came from South Africa. He was an officer with the King's African Rifles. He was also a married man (married to someone other than Mum's mum, that is). Mum's mother was 17. She was obviously as gullible as 17-year-old girls usually are.

When Mum was born, a notice was put in a number of local papers asking for someone to care for a newborn girl. The woman who became Mum's 'Nana' read the notice, exclaimed 'poor bairn!', and so Mum spent her first eight years in South Shields, County Durham.

It was, apparently, a magical childhood. Mum and her 'brother' Matt used to tumble out of bed, throw on shorts and hurtle down the cliff path to the beach, where they'd spend the day. At weekends they would take the Tyne ferry to visit Nana's sister. Nana's husband was a ferry pilot, and Mum basked in the status this gave her.

When Mum was eight, her mother married. Mum's new step-father, Teddy, was a man in a million. Mum adored him. But she did not appreciate being torn from her life in the north. She hated London, where no one could understand a word she said. She was told her father had died in the war. She felt betrayed when she learned the truth.

But it was her mum, not her dad, who she believed had betrayed her.

I never shared Mum's feelings about her dad. My thoughts were always for his wife, and for the 17-year-old whose life he might have ruined.

But he can't have been all bad. At least he kept in touch. Mum even met him. She only had hazy memories of having tea with 'Uncle Richard', but how poignant these memories became once she realized …

How she longed to discover more about her beloved

father. So it had always been her dream to go to South Africa. Before we went I did some homework, discovering where Mum's dad had lived, worked and was buried. I wrote to the people living in his old house, hoping we might visit. But they didn't reply. I also wrote to the cemetery where he was buried, but we could find no trace of his grave.

But this was all one to Mum. She was finally in South Africa, finally breathing the air breathed by her beloved dad. It was worth conquering my fear of flying to see Mum's delight in achieving this dream.

What matter if now she remembers nothing of it?

Our South African holiday was completely fantastic. The holiday company (Saga), told about Mum's coeliac disease and her Alzheimer's, dealt with everything admirably. The group was great fun and Mum was adopted as a sort of mascot (this was always happening to her). I'd heartily recommend Saga's holidays.

Perfectionism

Christmas! A perpetual reproof. Every year I intend to have finally learned how to use mail merge, have all my addresses typed so I can print off labels, and have all my Christmas cards (bought in the January sales) ready to go at the press of a button.

I intend to have been a one-woman production line of festive truffles, mince pies, brandy butter and other goodies, all beautifully wrapped in shiny paper (also bought in the January sales) and dispensed with serene smiles.

My tree will be up and decorated in plenty of time, surrounded by parcels properly labelled and chosen with the recipient especially in mind.

But every year the ghastly truth: I cannot get my act together.

My tree is up (that's not bad, is it?). But every post brings an avalanche of cards, serving only to remind me that I haven't even bought mine. As for having typed my addresses into my computer … no chance!

Yet this year, without Mum, I thought it would all be so easy.

Mum's nursing home has been ready for Christmas for weeks. There is a multi-coloured tree in every sitting room, cards galore and carols blaring from every speaker. Mum even said 'Happy Christmas' to me yesterday. The noticeboards are full of events to which relatives are warmly invited, and on Christmas Day there will be the full works.

I shan't be going to lunch itself. I shall be with the friends with whom I always spend Christmas. But I am going to just about everything else, starting tonight when a group of carol singers from a local school is coming.

It's good, of course, that local schools and organizations remember people like Mum at Christmas, though I wish they'd remember them at other times, too. The home does its best – generally pretty good – to ensure that residents are kept active and happy, but inevitably they spend a lot of time sitting and staring.

If local schools and churches were each to put on some form of entertainment for one of the local nursing/residential homes once a month, that would go a long way towards making such homes *a part of* the local community, instead of *apart from* the local community. The Brownies, Cubs, Scouts and Guides could get involved, too. It would be good for everyone.

I would organize it myself, but the belief I have time to do this is precisely the sort of belief I need to drop. Sometimes I even think – ludicrously – that the whole point of Christmas is to puncture my fond belief that I can do everything.

Imperfection has its consolations, of course … if I were perfect I wouldn't have any friends to whom to send cards.

> I *still* haven't put my addresses on computer. But I have
> found someone who does labels for me, for £50. Expensive?
> Perhaps. But my goodness me it's worth it. If only I had
> known about it when Mum was living with me.

Love

Sometimes being with Mum is so life-enhancing I feel buoyed up
for hours. It was like that the other night.

The evening didn't start well. Some students were coming to
sing carols. So everyone was walked or wheeled into one of the
sitting rooms. With about 50 residents, staff, relatives and a lot
of wheelchairs, it was a bit of a squeeze. But Mum was in a fine
mood and happy to be asked several times to move for someone
else.

The students arrived and walked self-consciously into the
space left for them. They launched into 'Hark the Herald Angels
sing'.

Mum was electrified. Slowly she got up and moved towards
the choir. I considered stopping her but she wasn't doing any
harm so I followed. She walked into their midst and stood
transfixed with wonder. At the end of the carol, she looked at
them, then at me, then at them again. Then she said 'Oh, I *love*
you, I love you, I love you *all*.'

When they resumed Mum sang along with them. She
couldn't remember the words, of course. But she had the tune
bang on. Her voice is still lovely.

As is her smile. Toothless, but so expressive of love and
pleasure that I felt quite tearful. I doubt the choristers will ever
feel as appreciated as they did that night. My heart almost burst
with love and pride.

During the interval we sat down. When the singing restarted

the man next to me, a new resident, started crying. I put my arm round him, held him tight, and asked if he was OK. It took a while to understand his mumble. But it became clear that his tears were of pleasure, not pain. He was just as overcome as Mum.

Dementia is often portrayed as dehumanizing. To the extent it destroys the capacity to reason, this is right. But the capacity for reason is only one of the things that manifests our humanity. Dementia is very far from destroying the other: the capacity to love. The other evening Mum and the gentleman next to me demonstrated their humanity in spades.

Yesterday I went to a musical afternoon at the home, hoping for the experience to be repeated. It was not to be. Mum was asleep in a chair. So were most of the other residents.

Naturally great efforts were put in to rouse them. It is very disappointing when you want someone to be jolly and they won't go along with it. But when one resident, a woman who hardly ever speaks, suddenly yelled loudly and clearly 'Shut up!', we allowed our efforts to subside.

Oh well, some you win, some you lose.

What a magical evening this was. Just remembering it makes me smile. To think that only six months before this, our life – Mum's and mine – had been so difficult I had even wondered whether to act on her oft-expressed wish to die. Mum's nursing home was, for her and me, a real life-saver.

Joined-up Thinking?

Did you see the Government's announcement that it intends to train GPs to look for early signs of dementia in their older patients?

I have mixed feelings about this. It will raise awareness of dementia, which is good. But what on Earth does the Government intend to do about those who, as a result of this, are diagnosed with dementia earlier than they might have been?

After all, in its wisdom the Government also announced recently that the only drug available to those with early dementia – Aricept – is too expensive to be provided on the NHS.

Is this what passes for 'joined-up thinking'?

I remember when Mum was first diagnosed. Actually, no, I don't remember this. The diagnosis for some reason was given to my younger brother. He decided not to upset anyone with the information. (I have asked this question before, but what on Earth *does* one make of brothers?)

But I do remember the consultant talking to me about 'the diagnosis', and the hollow in the pit of my tummy when I asked her to explain.

A diagnosis of dementia is – er – a real downer. At least in 1999 Mum was given Aricept, so we felt we were doing something. But even so, Mum plunged into a deep depression from which, oddly enough, she emerged only as the dementia started to bite. This enabled her to go into a decent state of denial.

It would have been far better, to my mind, if she hadn't been told at all.

On the other hand, it was better that the rest of us knew (notwithstanding Richard's protective instincts). At least it meant we could start planning.

But planning *what* exactly? There's little chance of being accepted at a residential home once you have a diagnosis of Alzheimer's. They will take people who are simply forgetful, but they double-lock their doors against anyone with a diagnosis.

So this leaves you looking at nursing homes that admit patients with Alzheimer's or other forms of dementia. But there are few things more frightening, if someone you love has just been diagnosed with dementia, than looking around such a place. Even Mum's lovely home takes a strong stomach if you are unused to dementia.

I was able (and willing) to bring Mum to live with me. But I am the last to say that everyone should do this. I was very lucky in the relationship I had with Mum. And anyway, few people have lives that make taking on an elderly parent, especially one with dementia, feasible.

Wouldn't it have been better for the Government to sort out how to care for those with a diagnosis of dementia *before* training GPs to make such diagnoses earlier?

> Whenever committees of the great and the good are asked to pronounce on the expected explosion of dementia in the relatively near future, I always cast my eye down the list to see whether carers are represented on the membership. Often they are not. It makes me want to SPIT!

Weight Loss

I arrived as they were serving supper last night. It was a lamby-tomatoey thing, with rice. It looked delicious. So I had some. It *was* delicious. So I had more.

The staff love it when relatives eat with residents. They believe residents eat more. In Mum's case this might be true: yesterday she ate as much as I did. Then she had peaches and cream.

It is lovely to see Mum's appetite back. With a vengeance! Over the holiday I often went in for afternoon tea: always a mug of tea, served with a delicious fattening treat. Last time it was apple strudel, the time before a lighter-than-air raspberry sponge with cream.

As a coeliac Mum can't eat such things (I can and do). But she doesn't miss out. Once last week, for example, she had three *humungous* slices of gluten-free chocolate and date cake. She ate the lot. Made short work of it, too. She also made short work of her tea. Then she asked for another.

When Mum lived with me I worried about how little she drank. She'd have half a cup of coffee with breakfast, a cup of tea in the afternoon, and maybe one glass of water. She'd gracefully accept other drinks, but invariably left them.

But now! When I am helping her with supper I am constantly pouring out yet another drink for her. Last night she had four glasses of Ribena, smacking her lips over each, saying, 'This is nectar, simply nectar!' Mum always says this when she likes a drink; she's nothing if not appreciative.

Could it be that the temperature is so high in the home? Perhaps, but it is not noticeably higher than I used to keep the house (Age Concern recommended 21°C/70°F).

But one thing puzzles me: Mum is not putting on weight. Her legs are still little more than sticks, and her once magnificent bosom is now hardly noticeable (partly because they've obviously given up on bras, so her bosom is no longer where it used to be).

Perhaps Mum only eats a lot when I am there? If so, my guess would be that this is because I cut things up for her.

I recently went in to find her (and others) forlornly spearing some thick slices of beef. No way could they have eaten these unless they were cut into manageable pieces. The carers (always fewer on a Sunday) were busy feeding those who need feeding. Might Mum and the others have ended up eating nothing at all had I not arrived?

Hm. Worrying isn't it? I have had a word with the director of the home, and she has promised to look into it.

Mum's home was lovely ... but how could they have not considered the fact that people like Mum and the other residents would have trouble with such huge thick slices of beef? That's why it is important that if your piglet goes into a home you go in at mealtimes for a bit.

Cat Dementia

Do cats get dementia?

I ask because Fatcat is definitely displaying some symptoms. She is driving me potty.

For one thing there is her piteous mewing. It starts the minute she sees me and never stops. 'Meow!' she says, 'meoow! meoow! Meeooow! MEEEOOOW!'

AAArrgh! This so reminds me of Mum's constant repetitions.

Then there is the fact that, as with Mum, I can't move without Fatcat following me. Not only does she follow me, she gets under my feet. Literally under my feet; I can't move without standing on her paws or her tail. And whenever it happens she lets out the most terrible wail. I'm sure the neighbours think I am ill-treating her.

The irritation of this is exacerbated by the length of Fatcat's claws. As she walks on the wooden floor they click-clack like two pairs of high heels. It has the effect on me that the tick-tocking of the clock inside the crocodile had on Captain Hook.

Whenever I sit down she sits at my knee pawing me constantly and butting me with her head. She is the most demanding cat I ever met. I can't believe I once thought this of Oedipus.

As for poor old Oedipus … he can't put his head out of my bedroom without getting his ears boxed. Fatcat has always been a bit of a bully, but now she's a true despot.

In fact the only time she leaves me alone is when she is stalking Oedipus.

Oedipus goes past, minding his own business. Fatcat tenses, then silently creeps up on him. Then she leaps, her paws boxing at him viciously.

Oedipus responds in kind and the yowling has to be heard to be believed.

Given half a chance Fatcat would do away with Oedipus. This is probably because Oedipus sleeps in my bedroom. Fatcat has definitely got the message that she is *not* allowed in my bedroom. This doesn't stop her nosing the door open, peering in forlornly, or staring malevolently at Oedipus.

I have been trying to get rid of her, really trying. I have scoured the web and rung or e-mailed every cat rehoming place within a reasonable distance. But either they say there's no call for a cat as old as Fatcat (13), or that there's a waiting list a mile long. That is, if they return my call at all.

I think I might have to put her in her basket, take her to one of these places and simply leave her there, insisting that I cannot keep her any longer. They all say they would never allow a healthy cat to be put down.

But maybe Fatcat isn't healthy? Maybe she really has got cat-dementia?

A friend of mine, Sue, uses the RSPCA's 'Home for Life' service. You give them a donation, then if anything happens to you, they either rehome your cat or keep it safely in one of their homes. See the Resources chapter for more about Home for Life.

Direct Payments Revisited

Nine months before Mum went into her home, the Council granted me Direct Payments of £403 per week.

I was at breaking point. The Direct Payments were supposed to help. It was the Direct Payments, though, that broke me.

Anyway, with Mum settled, I wrote to the Council, asked them to stop the payments, audit my accounts and take back the £4,000 still sitting in my account (because of my fear of spending the money during the two-month lag between the payments being awarded and actually starting).

The payments stopped (useful proof they'd received my

letter). But nothing else happened. So £4,000 of Council money has been doing nothing in my account for six months.

A month ago I had reason to speak to the head of Social Services. So I mentioned this sorry story. Well! See what going to the top gets you. Almost immediately I heard from the Direct Payments team.

Not just from the go-fers, either. Oh no. I got an e-mail from the chap in charge. He suggested a meeting so he could tell me what was going on.

I immediately thought, 'Oh dear, he's going to try to convince me how wonderful the system is, when what I want is to tell him how and why, for me at least, the system didn't work.' I e-mailed him to that effect (more politely, I hope). He assured me he wanted to hear from me.

But he didn't. His enthusiasm for the Council's work on Direct Payments was palpable. He is totally committed to it. Wonderful he makes it sound. They're going to change this, re-jig that, re-brand this and make sure of that. It all sounds just dandy.

By nature I am the very opposite of cynical. But having been a carer for nearly 14 years I have been through several 'new dawns'. I haven't seen one of them change things for carers, except at the edges, and then often negatively.

It's not that the new ideas are no good. If they were actually implemented, competently, consistently, fully and within sensible time scales, they would make a huge difference. But they are often not implemented at all (because another new initiative arrives hot on the heels …). If they *are* implemented it is at break-neck speed, so those actually implementing them can't even wrap their minds around them, never mind their practice.

I find enthusiasm enormously appealing, but I wasn't convinced.

But here's something impressive: last night a man from the Council arrived (by appointment), took away everything relating to Direct Payments, and promised to sort them out for me!

Now *that's* service!

> The words 'new initiative' strike fear into my heart. It is
> not that new initiatives, especially those that might help
> carers, are not needed, it is rather that so many of them are
> all but useless to those of us on the ground. Lots of them, for
> example, simply turn out to be reorganizations. Upheaval
> for nothing (or at least nothing for *us* or our piglets.)

Guilty Feelings

In Mum's home there's a book for recording arrivals and departures. I am sometimes shocked to see it's two or three days since I visited Mum.

You might ask why this should bother me: Mum neither knows nor cares whether I visit. She can be sublimely indifferent to my presence, or even make it clear that she'd rather I wasn't there. So why should I feel guilty for missing a few days?

Interesting question, that. In fact the whole question of guilt and caring is interesting. Because of my proximity, I am the only person to visit Mum regularly. How come the one that does most visiting feels the most guilt?

But I feel less guilt now than I did when Mum lived with me. Then I felt constantly guilty. Probably because I was constantly aware of everything I wasn't doing.

Why, though, couldn't I have banished the guilt by reminding myself of what I *was* doing? Again, why should the one who does the most also feel the most guilt?

This guilt haunts nearly every carer. As a carer you never feel you are doing enough. And however serene you appear, you cannot but be guiltily aware of the ever-present fear you might explode.

It comes back to responsibility. If you are a carer, then unless you are able to convince yourself you are doing everything you can, you will feel guilt. But who *can* take responsibility for the health and happiness of another human being, and really convince themselves they're doing everything they can?

I gather it's the same with children. But children soon (well, eventually!) start taking responsibility for themselves. Piglets usually go the other way.

But which comes first – the guilt or the caring? Did I take on responsibility for Mum because I felt guilty? Or did I feel guilty because I had on taken responsibility for Mum?

For me it was the former. So the guilt was there first and can't have been caused by taking on responsibility for Mum. Or at least not by the decision formally to take on responsibility for Mum (one of the few Mum-related things for which I feel no guilt at all).

It seems to me that the guilt that is so much a part of being a carer comes back to love. If you love someone who becomes unable to care for themselves then you will feel responsible for them, whether or not you formally take on responsibility for them. Guilt comes with that sense of responsibility.

Tough, isn't it?

But when you're next overwhelmed with guilt, try congratulating yourself on your capacity for love, and remember what you are doing, instead of beating yourself up for everything else.

> Don't set yourself up for disappointment by expecting your piglet to be pleased to see you when you visit them in their home. Sometimes they'll be touchingly delighted. Mostly they will be indifferent. It might be useful consciously to accept that you visit for *your* sake, not that of your piglet.

Teething Problems

I went to see Mum yesterday. But my main aim was not so much to spend time with her as to see the director. I had a complaint. Or at least a question.

A few days ago, noting one of Mum's plants was dry, I put it to soak in the hand-basin in her bathroom. The following day it was still there.

Oh dear. Hadn't Mum's hand-basin been used for 24 hours? Hadn't her hands been washed after she used the loo? Hadn't her teeth been brushed?

The director, a lovely woman, saw me immediately, heard me out and promised to make enquiries.

Today she told me the result: apparently because Mum often needs a 'full wash' in the morning, she is usually taken to the main bathroom. This means that her bathroom doesn't get used. That explains why no one noticed the plant.

But on her teeth there's bad news. They do indeed often go unbrushed: Mum will neither brush them herself nor let anyone else do it. So rather than end up in a fight (which they certainly wouldn't win), the staff often just let it go.

Hearing this brought back the hassle I used to have with Mum's teeth. Wouldn't you think that an action performed twice daily for 80 years would have become second nature? But not the brushing of teeth. Not for Mum, anyway.

My goodness, I remember how she was with me as a child. There was no chance *whatsoever* I would get away without cleaning my teeth. Similar sternness was the only way, once the tables were turned, to get her to clean her teeth. She complained every time she did it. But she still did it.

Surely this is the only way you'll ever win on things like this? It is only by refusing to give in *ever* that you will convey the message you need to convey: that there is no point in making a fuss so you might as well get on with it.

Letting Mum off even once would therefore have started the rot (probably literally): why do something you don't want to do when snarling at someone will get you off the hook?

I don't blame the staff. Mum snarls well. Also it's easier to stick to your guns when you are the sole carer: who, after all, is going to suffer if you give in?

But now we are storing up big trouble.

One of my brothers suggests Mum's remaining teeth should be taken out before the trouble starts. But my feeling, and that of my other siblings, is that we should leave them alone unless and until the trouble starts. (Anyway, imagine trying to give Mum a general anaesthetic, and explaining the pain to her afterwards.)

Is any dentist reading this? Do you have a solution?

> I wish, when Mum first went into the home, I had insisted that they insist that she brush her teeth twice daily. At that point it would have seemed normal to her. By now it was too late and crossing our fingers was the only realistic action. Perhaps you know differently? Please let me know if you do (see Resources chapter for how to reach me).

Hugging

I have discovered a new way to make Mum smile. It's not completely new. It made her smile before. What's new is how often I do it.

It is giving Mum a series of ENORMOUS bear hugs. These are real arms-totally-round-her, our faces nestling in each other's necks so we can kiss each other, bear hugs.

This is something we have always done. But not ALL the time. But now there is so little I can do with or for Mum it's lovely to find something that works.

The first time I hug her she smiles. The second time (ten seconds later) she smiles again and her face starts to relax. The third time (another ten seconds) she starts to look like herself, and she says 'Thank you, thank you, that's lovely.'

I find this humbling. Why should Mum *thank* me for hugging her?

But I understand. Mum is lonely. Terribly lonely. Having advanced Alzheimer's is one of the most isolating conditions possible. It doesn't matter how much you want to communicate, the words just won't come. If, like Mum, being sociable has been so important, this must be incredibly distressing.

I discovered the efficacy of hugging when, because I'd been on my annual Lake District jaunt, I hadn't seen her for a week. When I walked in she was in the corner, thinner than ever, radiating gloom. She perked up a bit when she saw me, but she didn't really recognize me, even emotionally.

So I hugged her, long and hard. The effect was magic. So I did it again, and then again. Since then I have spent all my time with her giving her hugs. I swear it is doing her good.

It reminds me of something she said just after Dad died. I had said something about loathing the 'peace' bit in church where everyone hugs everyone else. 'Being hugged by strangers makes me shudder,' I told her.

'Well,' she said 'what you don't understand is how important it is to elderly people who don't ever get hugged. It's the part of the service I like best. It's the only time I ever get hugged these days.'

That shut me up. It also completely changed my view of 'the peace'. Now I go out of my way to make myself available to hug and be hugged. I try to be sensitive to any person who obviously feels as I used to (of whom there are definitely a few). But I positively seek out those who, like Mum, are starved of hugs.

If a simple hug can make someone feel so much better (and we all know it can), then I'm all for it.

Institute a 'hug routine'. Advance on your piglet with open arms, clasp them in a bear hug and *squeeze*, sighing loudly with pleasure. Sometimes you'll find yourself hugging a block of wood. But other times their face will light up as you advance and they'll join in with glee. Lovely!

All of Life Is Here

Mum was in fine form yesterday. Resplendent in her new pink pyjamas, she was obviously feeling chatty. We spent a happy 20 minutes talking nonsense. If Mum sounded as if she was asking a question, I answered a question. If she sounded as if she was telling me something funny, I laughed. If she seemed to be telling me something in confidence, I listened gravely and responded confidentially.

Such interactions can be extraordinarily satisfactory.

Mum is looking good, too. Her eyes are lively and expressive – even, in a funny way, aware, though aware of what there's no telling.

Yet I was so frightened of consigning her to a nursing home. It felt like such a defeat. I was sure she would hate it, that she would respond as she did the one and only time she went into respite care. I was prepared for tears, trauma and the most tremendous guilt.

But the time had obviously come. The same seems true of almost everyone who comes into Mum's home. I suppose it's partly because it only caters for those with very advanced dementia.

The whole place is like a madhouse. I suppose it *is* a mad-house. Literally. But I mean that in the fondest way possible. When I visit I feel I am face to face with humanity, and with what is important in life.

Oh dear, that sounds rather precious doesn't it? I'm sorry. But I mean it. In everyday life we are soothed by the social niceties into forgetting what is what. In Mum's home there are no soothing social niceties. The veneer of civilization is missing. All veils have been swept aside.

Last week, for example, I had to alert a carer to the fact that a dignified elderly lady had been caught short in the corridor and decided that there was no time like the present.

This is not an unusual occurrence. Carers need to be constantly alert. That elderly gentleman, rising in such stately fashion from his chair, is just as likely to undo himself, as take a walk. Mum celebrated my giving her a new pair of slippers the other day by peeing on them.

Most residents seem content, or even happy, but there are those who are not, and who demonstrate this frequently and loudly. One poor lady cries constantly. Another is permanently angry, and can be quite vicious. Another is constantly agitated, talking at you until, in self-defence, you have to turn away, despite the fact it feels so rude.

It is life in the raw. But it doesn't matter how damaged these people are, they are still human beings. Unlike the rest of us, they wear their humanity on their sleeves.

My day job is quite demanding, but anyone with the right qualifications could do it competently. But being able to make elderly demented people feel good about themselves really matters. Not so many people can do this. Thank goodness for those professional carers and nurses who devote their working lives to people like Mum. What would we do without them?

Newcomers

Mum's home is big. New people are coming into residence all the time. Most come with families.

New family members exude shock. Grim-faced, sometimes tearful, always anxious, guilt seeping out of them, it takes them a couple of weeks to settle. The new resident settles far more quickly.

It's not surprising, is it? You're not eligible for Mum's place until you are oblivious to where you are. But for families this is the moment of defeat.

Both my parents have been in homes. Both were moved suddenly. Rereading my blogs, it is obvious I wasn't entirely unaware of the looming of Mum's move, though equally obviously I was in denial.

With Dad it happened virtually overnight. One minute, so far as I knew from my twice-weekly telephone calls, Dad was fine. The next Dad was in hospital, having 'fainted' en route to the shops.

'No, you needn't come,' said Mum. 'He'll be fine.' But a week later it was becoming obvious from Mum's strained tone that he wasn't fine at all.

I went home. Dad was far from fine. He was never fine again. After three weeks the hospital insisted no more could be done and they needed the bed. Mum was beside herself. Then she bumped into a friend who recommended a home.

It was utterly the wrong place for Dad. He became convinced he was at school and that Mum was *his* mum, come to take him home.

Mum was traumatized. Three weeks later she couldn't bear it. She fetched his suitcase and took him back home.

For the next 18 months she cared for him, and I, as his Receiver under the Court of Protection [see pages 237–38 for more about what this means], cared for their money. My telephone calls increased to two a day (at least). My visits to one a month. Mum's voice went from controlled to desperate. Dad went from being Dad to being … well …

At one point I arranged for him to spend one day a week at a local nursing home so Mum had at least one day's break. It helped, but it was a sticking-plaster.

Then their doctor took matters into his own hands. He rang and said he had arranged for Dad to be admitted to the home he'd been going to once a week. I was horrified. But the doctor – to his great credit – was adamant. He wouldn't, he said, bet on Mum's lasting the month unless Dad was taken off her hands.

Ten years later, almost to the day, my doctor made the same decision about me (though I hope he wasn't worrying about my lasting the month).

Thank goodness for doctors who are prepared, when necessary, to overrule everyone else. More power to their elbow.

I don't think medics are given nearly as much training in dealing with dementia as they should be. All Mum's doctors were lovely. But I sometimes felt I knew more about dementia than they did. I certainly knew more about dealing with demented people. If the expected 'dementia explosion' comes as more and more of us live longer, this will have to change.

Pet-talk

The 'pet therapy' dogs were in today. Goodness, what a difference they make. There's an ancient golden retriever and a huge, black, curly-haired – er – dog. They are patience personified. Neither thinks anything of being man- or woman-handled, patted *very hard indeed*, or kissed repeatedly. I swear they smile.

Wolfie, the black dog, arrived as I did. I immediately felt cheerful. It's lovely to know I'll have something to talk about with Mum. She loves animals, especially dogs and horses. She loves cats, too, but cats would always have been trumped by dogs and horses, had either been practical.

Sure enough, Mum's face lit up as Wolfie walked in wearing his smart day-glo jacket. She stroked his silky ears, kissed his damp nose and entwined her fingers in his curly coat. He just sat there looking pleased and thumping his tail. They say fondling animals reduces blood pressure. I'm sure they're right.

Talking of fondling animals, I think I have found a home for Fatcat. Now that really *would* be something. Oedipus will be delighted. Poor Oedipus, not above bullying other cats himself, is cowed by Fatcat. She only has to look at him to have him fleeing for cover.

Now it comes to it, though, I find myself oddly reluctant to part with her. I have got used to her. Oedipus is a nasty-tempered animal who will allow himself to be fondled only on his terms. Fatcat adores being petted. Boy, can she purr. She is also, of course, a living link with Mum. Amazingly, I will miss her.

But she deserves better than I can give her. I complain about Oedipus not being an affectionate cat, but actually this suits me well. I haven't the time to devote to a cat who needs affection as much as Fatcat. The young couple who might take her clearly adore cats. I think even Fatcat will get petted enough.

There is one thing, though: this young couple live on a houseboat. Fatcat will be a boatcat! This rather threw me at first. Fatcat is 13. She never was the most adaptable of cats. How on Earth will she take to living on the water?

But she won't, after all, have much to get used to because she will be an indoor cat. Rather than risk her falling into the water, Tim and Poppy intend to provide her with an 'igloo' cat tray, and keep her inside. This will certainly meet Fatcat's approval. She *hates* going outside. Especially when it's cold. Apparently Tim and Poppy even have a conservatory. Fatcat will be able to sit on a cushion, soaking up the warmth of the sun's rays through the glass.

Fatcat heaven!

> The Alzheimer's Society produces a 'This Is Me' leaflet for carers to complete and give to nurses or carers if a piglet has to stay in hospital. It provides information about likes and dislikes, how they like to be addressed and an account of their interests. Phone the Society up (the number's in the Resources chapter) for a copy.

Sweet Treats

Mum is still in wonderful spirits. It is liberating to go in and find her teasing the nurses, or good-naturedly chattering animated nonsense to the old lady sleeping next to her. I go away completely guilt-free, indeed positively feeling good about her. To think that six months ago Mum was begging me to help her die.

Now my biggest problem is what to do about her constant need for handkerchiefs, and what I can take to her that will give her pleasure.

The former is not really a problem, I suppose. Not for me, anyway. When Mum needs to blow her nose, which is frequently (she always said this is a sign of good health), she just uses whatever she is wearing, the tablecloth, or a napkin. All these things go straight to the laundry at the end of the day, so what's the problem?

Well, every time Mum hikes up her jumper and blows her nose on it I cringe. It's even worse when she uses the jumper of the person next to her.

When she went into the home I supplied her with handkerchiefs by the dozen. But they've all disappeared. I took another lot recently. But Mum has forgotten what they are for. Anyway, the carers have better things to do than find Mum's handkerchiefs. It is pointless to replace them again.

It's a shame. I like taking Mum presents, and at least, in replacing the handkerchiefs – and the other things that go missing – I can pretend. But I do not feel that I am giving her a treat: Mum shows not the slightest interest in them.

Taking her flowers or plants has become equally pointless. If they register with her at all it is not obviously with pleasure. Mum has become oblivious to the finer things of life. Books are hopeless. Even the big picture ones she used to enjoy. I don't think even pictures have meaning for her now.

I can, of course, give Mum a hug or a conversation, but there is only one concrete thing I can take her that will make an impact: something sweet.

Mum never had a sweet tooth. Now she devours anything sugary. But by indulging myself in taking her such things, I am merely hastening the day when all her teeth will have to come out.

> Your visits will not be the nice, warm, chatty episodes pictured in the home's brochure. Your piglet might take your presence as permission to behave badly. They might sleep through your visit. They might look at you as if they've never met you. Or as if they hate you. Remember, it isn't personal.

Poor Fatcat

Fatcat is on the way out. I took her to the vet to get her claws trimmed. But I could see from the vet's sombre face that the news wasn't good.

Fatcat has lost half her body weight since she last saw the vet. I didn't think this was anything more sinister than Mum's not being there to feed her junk. I was wrong. She has a thyroid problem. It is causing her to lose weight, and making her heart work overtime. Poor old Fatcat's heart is about to give up. She also has a 'mass' in her tummy. It's a toss-up to see which gets her first.

Oh dear.

The vet suggested a blood test. There is a 'cheap' one (£69.90) or an expensive one (I didn't ask). Either would confirm the thyroid condition, perhaps tell us something about the mass and enable the vet to decide on the best treatment. I decided to go for the cheap one. But as I had forgotten my diary I couldn't book her in.

Then, on the way home, I thought 'Do I really want to prolong Fatcat's life?' There's no doubt Oedipus would say 'No.' I hate the way they constantly scrap with each other.

I have decided, therefore, to let Nature take its course. The vet confirms that Fatcat is still a happy cat, and I will do what I can to keep her happy until the end. But I shan't postpone the end.

I do wonder, though, if I am doing the right thing by Mum. Mum, I'm sure, would have done anything – short of letting Fatcat suffer – to keep her alive. Fatcat's insurance policy testifies to that: it exists because Mum once spent £900 (£900!!) to set a leg that Fatcat broke leaping out of a tree. Horrified, I got Fatcat insured. Naturally we've not used the policy since.

I could use it now.

But since Mum has been in the home she hasn't even mentioned Fatcat. I like to kid myself she enjoys my talking to her about Fatcat. But actually she just likes me to talk to her. Anyway, my doing this doesn't depend on the state of Fatcat's health.

When Maive, Mum's best friend, died I told Mum about it. It was very moving. I swear Mum took it in. Her actual words were 'Thank you for telling me.' It was probably the most lucid conversation Mum and I have had since she went into the home.

But I don't see I have anything like the same obligation to tell Mum about Fatcat. If Fatcat is in Mum's memory at all, I shall let her stay there as a young and faithful companion.

> It is worth spending some of your valuable time on finding out if you are doing everything you can to maximize the pension you will eventually get. You need to check that you are getting Carers credit if you are entitled to it, or Home Responsibilities Protection. Contact the Pensions Advisory Service (see the Resources chapter) on 0845 601 2923 for free impartial advice.

Deterioration

Mum was in a foul mood the other day. She said 'No' to everything, bared her teeth and snarled when I tried to hug her, and generally made it clear she wanted me to go away.

One of the carers told me she'd tried to do Mum's hair and Mum had punched her. This mood used to herald a developing UTI (urinary tract infection). But yesterday Mum was OK, though not exactly cheerful.

I think Mum is deteriorating further. If she had stroke-induced dementia I'd say she had gone down a step. She's definitely not where she was even a couple of months ago.

She no longer understands anything. Even the simplest command ('lift your foot') goes over her head, and her own command of language has disappeared. Like a child she now puts everything into her mouth. I took her some flowers for Mother's Day, and before I could stop her she'd bitten the head off one of the daffodils. If I hold her hand, she'll try to suck my fingers.

But someone has obviously succeeded in holding her hand.

For the last two weeks Mum has been sporting the most – er – striking nail décor: dark red nails, with silver half-moons.

I adore seeing someone has bothered to sit with Mum and do her nails. To do those particular nails someone must have sat with Mum for a while: they were meticulously done. Mum would have adored having someone's attention for that long.

But they started to look tatty quite soon. Not that this bothers Mum. Or me. But then it occurred to me that if I did her nails it would give me something to do with her.

So today I took in some nail-polish remover and a pale beige varnish of the sort Mum would have liked. It took me half an hour to remove the dark red. Then another 15 minutes to repaint them.

I'd kill for Mum's nails. They're beautiful: strong, oval and just the right size. Her hands used to be beautiful, too. But now they're so thin you can see every bone, especially as her skin is almost translucent.

They're also covered in lurid bruises. In fact she's got bruises all over her. It was always easy to bruise Mum. But these days you can damage her almost by looking at her. She doesn't have an ounce of protective fat.

Yesterday I walked behind her as she was taken to the loo. Her shoulder blades are painfully prominent. I could put my hands around the top of her thighs. She is fading away in front of me.

But according to the carer who tried to do her hair, she still packs one BIG punch.

Anything that involves physical contact is a good thing to do when you are visiting your piglet. Doing their nails or hair, giving them a facial, shaving them … So long as it is something they've done many times before, the familiarity of the process – and perhaps the emotional memory – may soothe them.

Love All

Now here's an interesting subject: the love lives of carers.

Bet that woke you up?!

Also bet any interest it piqued has been extinguished already. Love lives? How on Earth would a carer have a love life?

Many carers, for a start, are caring for their partners. I shouldn't imagine that does anything for their love lives. I was always thankful I cared for my mum. One expects to care for one's parents. To me it didn't feel unnatural that as I waxed, Mum waned and the roles changed accordingly.

Whatever the vows made in happier times, it must feel like a violation to care for someone who was once your partner, your equal, your helpmeet. I remember my friend saying, as she sobbed in my arms about the unfairness of her husband's dementia: 'And I must face the fact that my marriage is over.' She was 50.

I didn't know what to say. What could I say? Her marriage *was* over.

You don't have to be caring for a partner, though, for caring to ruin your love life.

How does one juggle the demands of a partner (and children?) against the demands of one's piglet? Hard enough if the partners are caring for their child. At least they're in it together. But how do they ever find the time, never mind the energy, to have fun together?

If one of the partners is caring for a parent, this must get worse. My decision to bring Mum to live with me was unilateral: I wasn't foisting her onto a partner. However supportive one's partner, the guilt endemic to caring must be magnified 100-fold by involving someone else. Again, how does one go from providing the most basic of personal services to one's mum or dad, to being a sexy playmate for one's partner?

When I brought Mum to live with me, I didn't have any of these difficulties to negotiate. Not having a partner has its advantages. Anyway, what on Earth would I have done with a partner when by 8 p.m. I was completely exhausted?

But now Mum has been in her home for six months. Life is coming together for me. I am finally sleeping through the night, finally shopping for one instead of two, and finally relaxing back into my real self, after 14 years of worry and stress.

But now I am feeling good. Very good.

Apparently I am looking good, too. I have had so many compliments lately that I am beginning to feel very attractive. Yesterday my cousin asked me if I had a secret lover to explain my 'sparkle'.

The answer is 'No.' But goodness, what an exciting thought!

> Internet dating sites are a godsend for carers. If only the very fact of being a carer weren't such a turn-off. What carers need, by way of lovers, is other carers. Actually, thinking about it, it is quite a good way of quality-controlling potential lovers: anyone prepared to care for another person can't be all bad. Check out the carers' chat zones.

Ominous Diagnosis

The other day Mum's home called to say that Mum had a temperature. They were going to give her paracetamol and call the doctor. Later they rang to say that her temperature had gone down, and that the doctor hadn't found anything wrong.

I saw Mum that evening, and apart from the fact that, try as I might to persuade her, she wouldn't eat anything, she didn't seem too bad.

The following day I again went in at supper time to try to encourage her to eat. Mum did not seem at all well. She was very sleepy, and every time she moved she appeared to be in pain. I rang the doctor, to discover that Mum hadn't allowed the doctor to examine her on the previous visit, so it wasn't surprising she found nothing. I asked the doctor if she'd please visit again.

A few hours ago I spoke to the doctor. The news is not good. Mum has a 'mass' in her right bowel.

That word 'mass'. It's so ominous, isn't it? I keep thinking of the fact that that's what Fatcat has, too. But this thought seems oddly irreverent, as if I am comparing how I feel about Fatcat to how I feel about Mum.

But what do I feel about Mum? I feel numb. I feel wobbly. My hands, as I type this, are shaking. I also feel an odd sort of excitement.

Goodness, that sounds terrible. But I have been expecting something like this for so long that its arrival is almost a relief.

As the doctor pointed out, though, it could be something as simple as stools. The only way of finding out would be to take Mum into hospital for a scan or an x-ray.

But that would agitate Mum beyond belief. And for what? If they do find a 'proper' mass (as the doctor put it) what are we going to do, subject Mum to a general anaesthetic and a stay in hospital?

I don't think so.

Thank goodness I have Mum's 'Living Will', which explicitly asks that she be 'allowed to die' should there be no reasonable prospect that she would recover from an illness that would cause her 'severe distress' or render her 'incapable of rational existence'.

But the family might disagree, and obviously this is a decision we must take together. I am waiting to hear from them.

In the meantime I am comforted by the fact that yesterday, when I was stroking Mum's hair and telling her she was beautiful, she looked me straight in the eye and uttered a whole sentence: 'You're a very nice person,' she said, 'sweetie-pie'.

It's bringing the tears to my eyes to think about it.

> If you're in need of money, see if you can get a one-off grant from the Council, the Carers' Centre, the Alzheimer's Society or any other charity in your area. You'd be amazed at the number of little pockets of money. They gave me £400 once.

The End of the Chapter

Last Wednesday I spent two hours with Mum. I had intended just to hug her. But I was still there when supper started. So, hoping to persuade her to eat, I stayed.

She managed five teaspoonsful of ratatouille. But her heart wasn't in it. I was ridiculously proud, however, when she then ate two small flapjacks.

She didn't seem to be in pain, though she clearly wasn't comfortable. At about 6.15 she was getting sleepy, so I gave her another hug and left.

At 12.45 a.m. I almost fell out of bed when the phone rang. It was the home. Mum had been vomiting. They wanted me to confirm I didn't want an ambulance. I confirmed this, and said I was coming.

For 20 minutes I couldn't do anything right. I was half asleep but every fibre of my being was directed at Mum. Finally, no underwear, my jumper inside out, my shoes only just on the right feet, I went to get my bike. Only to remember I'd left it in town.

I had to walk. It was a full hour later that I punched in the home's security combination and rushed to Mum's side.

She was asleep. But as she had vomited twice, a couple of hours apart, I decided to stay. The nurses found me a mattress, and I changed into a pair of Mum's pyjamas. I lay on the mattress, listening to the sounds of a nursing home at night, and mentally packing myself a bag for a protracted stay.

Then Mum started making little whimpering sounds. Half an hour later she was clearly in pain, and the doctor was called again. But when she arrived, she had no morphine. She gave Mum an injection of something else and assured me it would take effect in about half an hour.

Half an hour later Mum was in agony. And so was I. Is there any torture more exquisite than to see someone you love in pain, yet be unable to do anything?

Throughout the night I had been wondering whether I should ring my sister and brothers. But Judy and Richard were abroad. It seemed cruel to ring them when they couldn't do anything until the following day. I did ring Christopher, having forgotten that without a car he too would be helpless.

At about 4.30 a.m., Mum abruptly stopped writhing. She lay on one side breathing heavily, her eyes open but not seeing. I hope she was feeling and hearing because I was stroking her and telling her how much I loved her. Then her breathing slowed and became intermittent.

At 5.30 a.m. on Maundy Thursday, my darling Mum drew her last breath and died.

You might want to check with your piglet's nursing home that they are prepared for an emergency such as this. I was beside myself with anguish during the hours Mum was in pain and no sensible pain relief was available.

Mourning Mum

After Mum died I sat with her for about an hour. Then I brushed her hair, gently washed her face and removed her wedding ring. My tears were falling freely. The two nurses who had shared the watch were wonderful, hugging me and assuring me Mum was at peace.

Then the strange realization that there was nothing more to be done. Feeling profoundly alone, I walked home.

My thoughts were everywhere. Snatches of Mum's terrible last night jostled with memories of happy times. So many happy times. I remembered her whooping joy when she graduated, her relish as she tucked into a huge knickerbocker glory, her triumph as she mastered the controls of a Vespa in Spain, her determination as she coaxed her car up an incredibly steep hill in the Lakes …

It was too early to ring people: on autopilot, I showered and breakfasted. Then I made the calls needed to send the news cascading down the generations. Such a huge family. So many people who loved Mum.

Then back to meet the doctor who was to certify death. Morphine *had* been available. But the locum didn't know. When I'm able I shall make sure no one else suffers like Mum for a locum's want of information.

Again I sat with Mum for a while. Many of the home's carers came to share their memories. It was touching for me to see how many people she'd touched. Marcus told me she had been singing along with him only days ago. Peter, tears streaming down his face, told me she'd make faces to make him laugh. Karen told me of her wanting to visit the seaside. We cried together and it comforted me.

Then I chose some photographs to put on the noticeboard: the home's customary tribute. I added the congratulations card that the Queen had sent to Mum and Dad on their diamond wedding anniversary, and an article on their elopement that Mum had herself written for *Saga*, around the time of their diamond wedding. Tearfully I chose the clothes she would wear for her final journey.

Mum's dying on Maundy Thursday was a blessing. For a few days I was able to do nothing. There was nothing I could do: even in the face of death, everything closes for Easter.

But as Easter finished the wheels again started turning. The flowers, letters, cards and e-mails started to arrive. Again I was touched that Mum had touched so many. I wrote to all the powers that be and to all Mum's old friends. Every now and again I rang someone I suddenly thought of who might not otherwise hear.

My siblings and I started to make arrangements for the funeral.

> If you are on a low income you can get help with funeral costs. Eligibility depends on your circumstances rather than those of your piglet. The grant you get if you are eligible will not cover the full cost of the funeral. But it will help. See the Resources chapter under Help with funeral costs, page 282.

The Funeral

Few people arrange more than two funerals. But no matter. Undertakers and vicars arrange hundreds. Discreetly they take charge and everything runs smoothly. (Mind you, have you seen how much they cost? They jolly well ought to run smoothly.)

The running order was easy. Mum had left strict instructions about hymns: 'Praise the Lord', 'The Day Thou Gavest' (also sung at Dad's funeral) and 'Love Divine'. Three hymns and four children, each of whom wanted to pay tribute, doesn't leave much time between the vicar's topping and tailing.

I did the Order of Service and photocopied it onto thin ivory card. The death notice went into the *Times* and the local newspaper in Mum and Dad's village. We agreed that people would come back to my place, 5 minutes' walk from the church, after the service.

There was a hiccup when we discovered that Ian, Mum's brother and his wife, Betty, so helpful over the years, weren't able to come. But they insisted we shouldn't rearrange. It'll be a good excuse for a get-together at a later date.

The morning before, my sister and brothers arrived. We prepared the house and garden, collected things that needed collecting, shopped, cooked, cried and laughed. In the evening we went through Mum's stuff. More tears. More laughter.

I slept very badly. When I did sleep it was only to dream that it had all been a mistake: Mum was still alive and I had to run around cancelling everything.

The day dawned sunny and fresh. I spent half an hour in the garden cutting her favourite flowers to put on her coffin. After some frantic last-minute preparations, we were all changed and ready as the hearse glided to a halt outside the gate.

Seeing the coffin for the first time was a shock, and the tears came. They came again as we walked into church. Mum's coffin was proudly carried by two sons and two grandsons. Four tall, handsome men. Mum would have adored that.

She would also have adored the fact there were about 65 people in church; people from all parts of her life, including many of those who helped care for her in her last years. The hymns were sung lustily, and the tributes read tearfully but with composure. Mum was carried out to the rousing strains of the Hallelujah chorus.

Immediate family went to the crematorium for the final rites: a dignified and solemn farewell to our beloved mum, now at rest.

Then back to the house, where about 45 people were eating, drinking and reminiscing in the glorious spring sunshine.

It was a good party. Mum would have loved it. I'm sure she was there in spirit.

I did with Mum exactly what I had done with Dad … went for the first undertaker I thought of. In each case it would have been more sensible to shop around. The price of funerals is horrendous. At Dad's funeral they offered 'pew cards' for those attending to complete. This was extremely useful afterwards. It is very difficult otherwise to remember who was there. I asked for them for Mum, too, but messages were mixed and it didn't happen.

Red Tape

For a few days after Mum's death I had some peace in which to start the process of assimilation.

But then the whirlwind started.

Death generates a huge amount of work, and I am not just talking about the funeral. The funeral was easy. It was therapeutic. It accorded precisely with my inability to think of anything but Mum. For the funeral all I had to do was think about Mum, but in a busy rather than a maudlin way. Just what I needed.

But since the funeral all this other stuff has descended. It is all Mum-related, but the winding up of a life doesn't involve reflection on that life so much as the marking of a life – the funeral – does.

Mostly it involves money and officialdom. Oh joy … my favourite things. It's amazing, in particular, how much money-related administration is generated by the death of someone who had no money.

Here's a tip – if you have Power of Attorney for someone who dies, get balances of the accounts you were administering *before* you tell them she's dead. If you tell them she's dead *then* ask for the balances, they won't give them to you. Typical, eh?

Another tip: get several copies of the death certificate. I seem to have sent off hundreds of them to all sorts of bods who have suddenly acquired an interest in Mum.

Interestingly, the Government came up trumps: I completed the form the registrar gave me, and that was it. Remind me of this when it is discovered Mum's pension wasn't cancelled after all.

Then there are the administrative narkies. You'd think I'd know whether Mum's maiden name had an 'e' or not, wouldn't you? But Mum herself was undecided – she used the two versions interchangeably. On her marriage certificate there's an 'e'. On her birth certificate there isn't. Her death had to be registered with both.

Then there are the tears.

But they're good tears. Healing tears. Tears of happiness as well as of sadness. Mum is dead. But she had a good life. She also had a pretty good death. Yes, there was pain at the end. But it could have been so much worse.

Most importantly, between us nothing was left unsaid or undone. I wear her wedding ring and feel her presence all around me. Love really doesn't die even if people do.

Next week I shall bring this blog to an end. For 14 years I have cared for my beloved parents. I must turn my attention elsewhere. But I think I have earned the right to a final reflection on caring and carers, and in my final blog I shall exercise that right.

Please join me!

> When you are ready you might like to use your experience as a carer to help other carers. The Alzheimer's Society has a peer support network through which experienced ex-carers help current carers. If this is the last thing you want to do, try some other sort of volunteering (see Resources chapter). You might of course feel like doing nothing at all. This is allowed!

The Final Saga Blog

I probably came to caring as you did. One minute I was living my life, the next I was enmeshed in the Alice in Wonderland world of Social Services, memory clinics, aids, appliances and assessments.

It happens every year to thousands of us. Out of nowhere we suddenly find ourselves doing an extraordinary and important job ...

... with no training, no preparation, no information, no 'career path' ...

... and for nothing, no thanks, no medals, not even any recognition.

My laptop insists 'carer' isn't even a word.

Becoming a carer is like falling through the looking glass: we discover a whole new world, one in which we must believe six impossible things before breakfast.

Why do we do it? Why do we put up with the sleeplessness, the guilt, the resentment, fury, helplessness, rage, hopelessness, misery and fear? Why do we not escape from the admin, the forms, the incompetence and the red tape? And from the jobsworths, petty bureaucrats and patronizing medics? Are we mad?

No. We know why we do it. If we're lucky it's because sometimes – just sometimes – we look at our piglets and our hearts explode with love. Or a stray word or look generates a memory that makes everything worthwhile. Caring can sometimes seem to be the only job worth doing. The only job that honours the things worth honouring.

Some of us aren't so lucky. I would not have been able to care from duty rather than love. But many of us do. If this is you, maybe you really are a saint? I salute you.

After 14 years of caring there's only one major thing I'd have done differently: I'd have arranged for Mum to go into a home earlier.

I was convinced only I could care for her. I was sure she would be unhappy in a home. I was wrong. A time comes when only demented people provide the right companionship for a person with dementia. A time comes when only professionals will do. A time comes when you must put yourself first. I shouldn't have waited until I hit a brick wall.

For a brief time Mum's home gave her a new lease of life.

If my saying this saves you from hitting that brick wall, I shall consider my work done.

There's so much else to say. But I have said enough. This is my final blog. I shall miss you. I am sorry I didn't respond to all your messages. Sometimes they were the only thing that made life worth living.

I hope to turn the blog into a book. I hope also to carry on speaking up for carers whenever and wherever I can.

Remember that if you feel you've been forgotten.

> You continue to count as a carer for one year after your piglet's death. This seems right to me. It will take you that long to stop thinking of yourself as a carer. Perhaps you might use this time to agitate on behalf of carers. Write to your MP, to your Council, to anyone else who will listen ...

The blogs that follow will bring you up to date on what has been happening since I finished the *Saga* blog.

The Joys of Driving

Shortly after Mum went into her home I started driving lessons. I wanted something to take me out of my comfort zone. Learning to drive would, I reckoned, help me forget everything about caring. Ridiculous, really; one doesn't stop caring because someone has gone into a home.

At 17 I also took driving lessons. I came to believe then that I wasn't a natural driver. I failed rather a lot of tests. Er ... five, actually. How embarrassing.

Then I lost interest. I always lived in either London or Oxford. In both towns cars are a liability. I had no children to provide an incentive. I didn't even think about it until Mum's going into a home left me with a vacuum to fill.

It mattered only once. In 1987 Dad had his first stroke. This was a decade before the stroke that took him down but not out. I was staying over for the weekend. I heard Dad shout from the bathroom. Then I heard Mum's voice, rising in panic 'Phil! Phil! Oh God, can you hear me, Phil?'

I rushed to them. Dad was on the bathroom floor. Mum was crouched beside him, her face a picture of anguish. Dad had clearly had a stroke. The left side of his face had collapsed. He couldn't use his left arm. I ran downstairs and rang the ambulance. It arrived within minutes.

But they would only let one of us travel with them. Shamefully, it had to be me. Mum had to follow in the car. The traffic was busy. Halfway there they decided to 'go blue'. I insisted they stop to tell Mum. Imagine her feelings, otherwise, on seeing them speed off, siren blaring?

Apparently, though, she nearly had a heart attack when they stopped to tell her.

This appalling experience didn't convince me to learn to drive. But being able to drive would have revolutionized my life as a carer.

Instead of having to trog Mum everywhere by bus, or pay for taxis, I could have ushered her into the car and driven her to the door. Instead of my stress levels being driven sky-high by special transport buses, and Mum having to sit for two hours at a time on the bus as everyone else was collected, I could have driven her to and from day care at a time of *our* choosing.

I could also have taken her for drives. We might have stopped off at the Little Chef and had her favourite garlic mushrooms. It would have been a reprise of my childhood when she took me for drives into the hills. Mum adored her car.

I passed my test, on the second attempt, two months after she died. I love driving as much as she did. As I journey through the countryside, I can feel her beside me.

Hubert, whose wife Phoebe has dementia, tells me you should resolve, before taking your piglet for a drive, to stay serene when your piglet releases their seat belt, your car goes berserk trying to tell you about it, and your piglet panics because the car is panicking. Reward yourself with an extra large sticky bun at the tea shop.

Getting Past It: Who, Me?

Denial. It is a wonderful thing. Mum was in denial throughout her dementia years. We never mentioned Alzheimer's. We talked about her memory being like a sieve, or so full that things leaked out … but dementia? Never!

This meant I had to fight Mum every step of the way at the beginning. She wouldn't have a cleaner (why did she need one?), or meals on wheels (that's for old people) and she categorically refused to give up driving (she'd *never* had an accident).

Every suggestion I was making was interpreted by Mum as 'You're past it.' But what could I do? She *was* past it.

Amongst the skills carers can put on their CV is that of extreme diplomacy.

It's not just piglets who go in for denial, of course. I denied how bad things were at almost every point in my caring career. Mum didn't want to know she was past it. I didn't want to know I wasn't coping.

The things that human beings can deny are legion. All men are mortal. But have you any idea how many people don't make wills? Some think that doing so is asking for trouble. Others are with Woody Allen: they think that in their case an exception will be made.

One thing human beings are given to denying is the possibility that they might one day need care. How else can we explain the fact that so many people are so reluctant to complete Lasting Powers of Attorney?

Well, I suppose it could be the money. Why they've made it so expensive I don't know. You can get them cheaper by going to paralegals, but care must be exercised if proper solicitors aren't used.

Anyway, I think the money is an excuse made by people who haven't understood what happens if you *don't* have an LPA. Actually, people don't want to give up control. They don't want to accept that it could become impossible for them – *them* – to look after their own affairs.

You can stress until you are blue in the face that until an LPA is registered a person is as in control as they have always been, and that if an LPA has to be registered it is not *having the LPA* that causes loss of control, but *the event that led to its having to be registered*. But still you'll find people resist.

My experience of being the carer of someone who didn't have one has made me an evangelist for LPAs. But I am used to the shifty looks people give me whenever I talk about them.

Why, after all, do *they* need an LPA? Only *other* people become mentally incapacitated.

> It is easy to persuade new carers that they should get an LPA for their piglet, but when you suggest they should have one, too, you are likely to be met with bemusement. In my opinion the carer needs one just as much as the piglet.

Hospital and the Demented

Recently I was knocked off my bike by a bus. It hit me from behind, leaving me unconscious face-down on the road.

The hospital was only 5 minutes away so the ambulance arrived quickly. I have a snapshot memory of racing through the corridors on a trolley. Otherwise I remember nothing.

When I came to I was on a backboard, my head restrained, an oxygen mask over my mouth and nose.

I was crying out that I was a carer and that Mum couldn't be left alone.

This was taken at face value until Felicity came in and told them Mum was dead. Poor Felicity had to decide whether to tell me Mum was all right or that she was dead. She chose the latter, thankfully. My memory started to return immediately.

I was fine (thanks to my cycle helmet, which was completely trashed). But I spent the night attached to a machine in the Clinical Decision Unit. I was next to an old lady with a nasty head wound. She had advanced dementia and was in great distress.

The nurses were doing their best. But they were clearly bemused and irritated by her repeatedly asking 'Where am I?' and her attempts to get out of bed. She kept getting hopelessly entangled in the bars and having to be heaved backwards. This did not relieve her distress.

My blood pressure must have been sky-high. I ached to help this lady, but was helpless. Luckily she was given something to make her sleep.

In the morning she was even more distressed. The ward was full. The nurses were being driven mad by the need to deal with her. I took myself off my machine and went to her. I held her hand and, pointing to my technicoloured eye, said repeatedly that she had one just the same, and that she was in hospital being stitched up. 'What a pair we are!' I exclaimed, over and over again.

It must have been obvious I was OK because the nurses left us alone. But eventually I had to get my broken thumb seen to. I have no idea what happened to her.

Why don't hospitals have on-call people who can deal with patients who happen also to have dementia? Such patients are hugely time-consuming for nursing staff. Their distress is distressing for every other patient. All this lady needed was someone to sit and reassure her.

Later I talked to the patient liaison service. I offered to set up such a service myself (perhaps my head *was* injured?). They thought I was complaining and became defensive. I gave up.

I think hospitals should have a team of volunteers on call to help patients like the old lady who was in hospital with me. Why, also, were the nurses so bemused by her condition? Were they simply overworked? Or were they not properly trained to deal with the demented? If not, this is going to be a big problem in future.

Fatcat's Swansong

About two months after Mum died I became aware that Fatcat was no longer a happy cat. She had begun yowling even more piteously than usual. She seemed desperate for food, but wouldn't eat anything. I rang the vet and described Fatcat's behaviour. Together we agreed the time had come.

Unable quite to believe what I was doing, I fetched the cat basket from the shed. I lured Fatcat into it with a kitbit (which she didn't eat). I drove her down the hill.

Carrying Fatcat into the waiting room, my knees started to wobble. I collapsed into a chair, Fatcat in her basket at my feet. The receptionists knew why I was there. They fetched me a glass of water. When I'd recovered they let us wait in a side room.

Then the vet called me in. We took Fatcat out of her basket and the vet examined her. She confirmed her telephone opinion.

She then explained the procedure and asked me whether I wanted to be with Fatcat whilst she had her injection. If not, she said, I could wait in the side room and she'd call me the minute it was done. Calling her assistant in, she assured me that she wouldn't act until I was ready.

By then the tears were pouring down my face. I felt quite faint. Fatcat and I were never the best of friends. But Fatcat was the apple of Mum's eye. Mum absolutely delighted in her. Fatcat returned the compliment. The vet and her assistant busied themselves at the computer, whilst I petted Fatcat and rubbed her head for the last time. I left the room, now sobbing quite openly.

Almost immediately I was called back in. Fatcat was lying on her side on the table. The vet hadn't mentioned that her leg would be shaved for the injection, and bits of her long fur were all over the table.

I stroked Fatcat's side as I watched the light die from her huge golden eyes. For 10 minutes I couldn't speak. All I could think of was that Mum was dead and now I was killing Fatcat. Again the vet, assistant now diplomatically elsewhere, was busying herself. She put no pressure on me to hurry. But after 10 minutes it was clear with Fatcat, as it had been with Mum, that life was irretrievably gone.

Carrying the now empty cat basket, tears still streaming, I paid the bill and returned to my car. How I manoeuvred out of that tiny car-park in such a state I'll never know. It was two days after I'd passed my test.

Later I comforted myself with the thought that Fatcat and Mum were staring adoringly into each other's eyes.

If you or someone you love faces losing a beloved pet, there is plenty of help on offer. The Samaritans have an animal bereavement arm; the Blue Cross run a counselling service. See the Resources chapter. You can also put 'pet bereavement' into Google and you'll find all sorts of help.

The Inevitability of Death

I was asked yesterday whether I missed my parents. The answer, if I'm truthful, is 'No.' I have two ways of explaining this apparently disrespectful attitude.

First, my parents' lives, and the way they brought me up, prepared me for their death.

I was never, for example, treated much like a child. Mum and Dad expected their children to be rational, sensible people. On the whole, we met those expectations.

This was consistent with a great deal of fun. With Mum in particular, laughter was constant. It was also consistent with the usual crises and instances of bad behaviour. It was a perfectly normal household. But it was one in which independence was encouraged and expected.

A serious question, for example, would prompt a trip to the library. Dad, or Mum, would help us think about where the answer might be found, then wait whilst we found it. I don't remember ever having anything I asked dismissed as unworthy. I do remember occasionally being irritated that they wouldn't just *tell* me the answer.

We were always encouraged to form our own opinions. If these weren't those of our parents, that wasn't a problem. I remember an election at which each of us supported a different political party. The house proudly displayed four different posters. Canvassers didn't know what to think.

It's possible we were given too much freedom. Although distressed when I was thrown out of school, aged 16, for truancy and disruption, they allowed me, five months later, to move alone into a bedsit in London.

The self-sufficiency my parents fostered in me has stood me in good stead. They would be disappointed if they felt they hadn't prepared me for their inevitable death.

Secondly, both my parents died when life had lost its point. Even if he was robbed of his last four years by emphysema, Dad's 84 years were mostly contented and productive. He didn't fail in any of the duties that meant so much to him.

Mum developed Alzheimer's ten years before her death at 89. Notwithstanding this, and the fact that – as you know – there were some very hard times during those years, when I look back at Mum's life I see she managed to wring from it, in her inimitable way, every last bit of enjoyment she could. She enhanced the lives of everyone around her.

It is in the nature of the human condition that life is finite. It is part of our human duty to accept this for ourselves, and to teach our children to do the same. In this task, as in every other, my parents succeeded admirably.

In writing this book I have tried to express the huge capacity for love nurtured in me by my beloved parents. If you have enjoyed it I'd love you to tell me so (see the Resources chapter for how to reach me). I continue to do everything I can to help carers. Remember you are not alone.

Marianne's Tips for Carers

Fantastic! *Saga Magazine* have asked me to list my tips for carers. I *hate* the usual anodyne tips: I'd happily 'take a break' and 'avoid stress': but *how*?

So I shall break the mould by offering ONE tip, and a guide to acting on it:

TIP: <u>IDENTIFY WHAT'S NEEDED TO MAKE YOU *YOU,* AND MAKE DAMN SURE YOU GET IT.</u>

Here's my guide to acting on it:

Step One: *List everything you'd really like to do daily, weekly, monthly and yearly.*

My ideal life includes a daily 20-minute walk, a thrice-weekly swim, a weekly outing with friends, regular theatre visits, occasional weekends away, a week's walking in the Lakes and two weeks somewhere hot.

Without these things I'd become resentful and irritable. Mum would feel vulnerable and I would feel guilty. Result: crisis.

But I work full-time and Mum, as you know, had advanced Alzheimer's and was living with me. How to achieve *any* of these things, never mind *all*?

Your wish list may be very different from mine. And writing it won't be easy if, like many carers, you can't remember who YOU are. Think about your 19-year-old self's dreams: then revive them.

Do not dwell on the barriers – if you do, you won't get anywhere.

Step Two: *For each listed item, say what you need to achieve it.*

For my wish list I needed: day care, respite care, time, willpower, substitute carers, hard-heartedness, extra funding, organizational skills and persuasive powers.

Day care allowed for the walking and swimming. But only if I exercised willpower to make time for myself.

This is probably true for you, too. If so then add 'time' and 'willpower' to your list.

For evenings out, the theatre and weekends away I needed substitute carers and a hard heart.

The last was non-negotiable. Mum got clingy when I had to go out. But should I have stayed in? It would only invite resentment. Unless you are naturally hard-hearted – unlikely, as you are a carer – it should be on your list.

You might be able to pay for substitute carers without extra funding. Even so, you might prefer to rely on people who do it for love (or at least guilt).

But then, like me, you will need organizational skills and persuasive powers, the former to decide when people are needed, the latter to get them on board.

The final part of working out what you need involves constructing a timetable.

Do you have exact dates when you'll want substitute care? Is anything entirely open (your walk?), fairly flexible (your swim, walking holidays?) or open until arrangements are made (outings with friends, theatre trips, weekends away?)?

Make your timetable of needs as precise as possible.

Step Three: *Brainstorm ways of getting what you need*

Some things on your list will be things you have to *be*. If you have trouble with willpower, prioritizing your needs, organization, persuasion or hardening your heart, then you need to work on yourself.

You could take classes (try your local Carers' Centre), read self-help books (try your library) or have coffee with friends and ask for tips.

Challenge any belief to the effect that you can't change – *why* can't you?

Getting substitute care will probably involve asking for help. This may hurt. I liked to think of myself as superwoman and hated asking for help. But for carers self-sufficiency is NOT WHERE IT'S AT.

List everyone who might provide substitute care. Include family, friends and neighbours, but be creative: the Guides, the church, local charities …? Might your local sixth form help as part of community service? Ask them. (In the early days I secured the help of several sixth formers who wanted to be doctors and thought it would look good on their CV.)

Order your list according to people's moral responsibility. Not so you can blackmail those at the top (though it's worth a try!), but so you can send a complete list (however rough) of when you need help, thereby giving a choice of dates and times.

This makes it easy for anyone who'd like to help, and difficult for anyone who doesn't. Anyone claiming to be unable to do *any* of your dates/times should be scrubbed off your Christmas card list.

Extra funding is available: the Alzheimer's society gave me £400, Age Concern provided a 'flexible friend', and my Carers' Centre gave 12 hours' free care. You won't get anything unless you ask. So ask.

You are entitled by law to day care and respite care. Do not be put off, as I was, by a Council employee telling you a carers' assessment is useless because there's no money. Exercise your rights.

Step Four: *Make an action plan*

If you were working to my plan, you'd need to visit the library, ring the Carers' Centre and arrange coffee with assertive friends.

You'd also have to contact family and friends, speak to neighbours and approach your local Guides/church/school.

In chasing funds you will be ringing many of those already listed: do not make two calls when one will do.

One of your first calls should be to your Council to sort out entitlements.

List everything you need to do, together with dates for doing it.

Step Five: *Implement the plan*

This one is easy – get on that phone!

Step Six: *Check your progress*

Every week I checked my progress over a congratulatory glass of wine: I was, after all, looking after myself as well as my Mum and that was A GOOD THING.

Step Seven: *Do not panic when things go wrong*

Sometimes people get flu, trains are late, and crises occur. Sometimes your piglet will refuse to play ball. Even the hardest heart has to melt sometimes.

The trick is to reflect on what's gone wrong, and on whether and how it can be righted. If it can be righted, plan and implement your strategy.

If it can't then just forget it …

… after all if, having acted on my tip, you are living roughly the life you want to live, then missing one treat is not the disaster it would be otherwise.

I hope this works as well for you as it did for me.

Carers' Fury

How are you?

I bet there's a good percentage of you who, if you answered this question honestly, would say: 'I'm FURIOUS!'

I'm not suggesting the rest of you are actively lying to me. I hope no carer is furious *all* the time. Maybe it is your day off. Some lucky carers might even manage *never* to be furious (*you* can stop reading here). But I suspect many carers feel compelled to keep their fury under wraps most of the time, because expressing it feels unsafe/unproductive/forbidden/not nice.

I understand this compulsion. Most of the time, expressing fury isn't productive. Yelling at an astonished milkman is not a good way to start the day. Snarling at the nice lady who has come to take your piglet for a walk is plain unfriendly. Snapping the head off the check-out girl will not secure good service (and why ruin *her* day?).

Many carers, of course, are female, and in our society I think females find it particularly difficult to express anger. But how do you do sweetness and light when inside you are *screaming?*

Sometimes fury is useful – it gives you the energy to fight. Carers need to fight. But only *some* of the time. Yet here you are furious nearly *all* of the time.

Some lucky carers have safety valves: understanding partners, supportive parents and/or siblings, rock-solid friends and neighbours; their price is above rubies. But it's totally understandable that we don't want to dump on them *all* the time.

But *why* are we so angry? Is there anything we can do about it?

Well, where to start on the 'why'? For every carer, the mix will be different. But the elements will be a combination of some (or all) of the following:

- infuriating jobsworths from the Council, the utility companies, the Social Services, the Inland Revenue, the Court of Protection, the Office of the Public Guardian, your broadband suppliers, the dispensing chemist …

- infuriating (and ungrammatical) letters from the Council, the utility companies, etc., etc. …

- all the inanimate things that are conspiring against you (the towel rail that fell off, the hand-held vacuum cleaner whose battery ran out, the washing-up liquid that chose to run out …);

- everything to do with your computer and its horrible ways;

- ditto the car and its unhelpful habit of needing to be filled up when you HAVEN'T GOT TIME;

- everyone's TOTAL lack of understanding of what you are going through;

- the behaviour of those who ought to be supporting you but aren't;

- the fact that your piglet's life is in your hands and you are SICK TO DEATH OF IT.

Hm. There is a distinction that might come in useful here. It is between 'immediate' and 'mediate' causes. The *immediate* cause of an event (an explosion of fury, for example) is whatever actually triggers that event. The *mediate* cause of an event might be quite different. It might be nothing more than the context needed for the immediate cause to do its work (the oxygen without which striking the match would have no effect).

QUIZ: FROM THE LIST ABOVE, IDENTIFY THE MEDIATE CAUSE OF YOUR EXPLOSIONS OF FURY.

That's right. Top marks. We carers wouldn't be the spitting, hissing bundles of fury we are (at least inside) were it not for the fact that our piglet's life is in our hands.

But there it is. Our piglet's life IS in our hands. There's nothing we can do about it. Over this we have no control. To express fury about it would be utterly and completely pointless.

It might also be dangerous. Yelling at the milkman is one thing. Yelling at our piglet is another. Around our piglet, iron control must be exercised. Otherwise, who knows what might happen?

Iron control must also be exercised around everyone who is helping you, or at least trying to help. No carer can do it alone. It takes a veritable army. There are the people from the day care centre, the special transport people, the mobility people, the memory clinic people, the care manager and everyone else at Social Services, the adult placement people, the chiropodist, the dentist, your GP, the receptionists at all these places, the neighbours, helpful family members ...

We are unendingly grateful to all these people. Without them our lives would be intolerable. So we spend our days saying 'Thank you,' 'It's so kind of you,' 'Would you mind ...?', 'Thank you,' 'Thank you,' 'Thank you.'

We mean it. Goodness knows we mean it. But day in, day out, we are thanking people for making it possible for us carry on doing something that makes us …

… *furious.*

Carers are springs coiled tight by the need to suppress themselves and express gratitude to others. We are on a hairspring trigger. Our triggers can be tripped by anyone or anything.

If you are like me, most of your expressions of fury go unseen by anyone but the cat. You haven't yet (I hope) actually thrown your computer across the room, but it has come close. The kitchen workbenches have felt the pounding of your fists on more than one occasion. The walls are used to being kicked. The cats have learned to scarper quick when you get started, and your language is *dreadful*. If you're not like me, you probably spend a lot of the time feeling guilty and apologizing.

All of us will occasionally lose our rags in public. You feel so *ashamed* when you remember your occasional outbursts against innocent people who got in your way on a bad day. You don't feel exactly sanguine when you admit to yourself that even the offences of some of the jobsworths weren't *so* dreadful.

But you are at your most helplessly furious when interacting with or thinking about those who – in your opinion – aren't pulling their weight. These people are nearly always family members. They might be partners, children, siblings or anyone else. They may not even be *your* family – the in-laws can be just as guilty. 'Caring destroys family relationships,' it should say on the packet. I have spent many a jolly evening with other carers roasting recalcitrant co-carers – *supposed* co-carers – over a bottle of wine.

Some co-carers sound as if they should be stood up against the wall and shot. Their behaviour is outrageous. Often this is just one person who, alone of their family, chooses to do nothing. Sometimes they don't even pretend to care.

But usually interactions are more subtle.

There are, for example, co-carers who help, but very much on their own terms. Yes, they'll take over for a week, but they're reluctant actually to commit to a specific week in which they'll take over. Yes, they'll be supportive, but not necessarily at the times you *need* support. Yes, they'll do things with your (joint) piglet, but not necessarily the things that need doing. Especially not *when* they need doing.

It's difficult to avoid the idea that the most important thing to these people (next to caring for your joint piglet) is to avoid giving you any grand idea to the effect that, just because you are the main carer, you are in any way in charge.

The opposite problem is posed by those who are willing to help, but who take no responsibility or initiative whatsoever. You must cook the suppers and leave them in the fridge/freezer. You must list the things that need doing, the times they must be done and instructions on how they should be done. This sort of person needs these lists on every occasion they lend a hand.

Then there are the co-carers who profess themselves more than willing to help. But who wait to be asked and, when asked, are too busy. The week you need help they are away on business. Or they are having a difficult time at work and can't spare the time. Or one of the children is desperately in need of support at school. They really *do* want to help, though, so don't hesitate to ring next time. These people never ring you.

The goal of these games seems to be to avoid giving you the impression that anyone is in charge *but* you. God forbid that they should be seen as an equal partner in this caring lark. Where would it ever end?

Whichever version plagues you, the subtleties of these interactions will not be lost on you. You will notice. Having noticed, you will have to decide what to do.

Unfortunately, you too are engaged in manipulative subtleties.

Oh yes, you are. Being a carer doesn't magically immunize you from family game-playing. Sibling rivalry, for example. All those little games you thought had been left behind decades ago? Lo! Here they are fresh, powerful and entwining you as securely as ever. Marital power plays? I don't care how long you have been married, you'll still be at it. Those feuds with the in-laws? Thought they'd been forgotten, did you?

Isn't there just a little bit of you, for example, that is triumphant that *you* are the main carer? Aren't you just a little cock-a-hoop that as the main carer you have the right – the *right* – to call the shots? Being on the moral high ground surely can't but give you just a tiny – tiny – thrill?

Just when you need to be at your most adult, it is as if you are dragged down into deepest, darkest childhood. Doesn't it just make you feel utterly, hopelessly, *helpless?*

No wonder you are furious.

At this point every carer needs, on their shoulder, a family mediator. Unfortunately, you have on your shoulder a furious child, egging you on into behaviour that is, to say the least, unhelpful.

The family mediator would whisper into your ear, 'Say firmly "I really appreciate your offer to help, but need to pin you down to some dates so I can book a holiday,"' Or they would urge you to state assertively, 'If you can't do 2 p.m., here is the number, would you cancel that appointment and book another?'

Instead, your furious child whispers: 'Ha! Here they go again. Typical. Of course they can't say when they'll come. Of course it's inconvenient. As usual they're leaving it *all* to you.'

So all that iron control you have been exercising elsewhere evaporates. All the gratitude you usually feel for anyone prepared to do anything at all for your piglet turns to fury. Here is a situation in which you can let go and do your VERY WORST.

Your worst will be some form of whatever it is your family

does in such situations. Perhaps you'll blow a fuse and enjoy a wonderful hissing, spitting, screaming, furious bout of rag-losing. Perhaps you'll turn on the ice, allow that dangerous tone to enter your voice and ring off with a farewell that would chill a brass monkey. Or perhaps your weapon of choice is sarcasm, so the rest of the conversation will consist of remarks intended to cut to the quick.

If you ever think I am setting myself up as an expert carer, or one who got everything right, please ask yourself how I happen to know all this.

If you have *never* acted in any of the ways described, go away, you're embarrassing me.

You can, of course, use different tactics at different times. Or you might engage in *all* these tactics. Either way, doing your worst can be – I'm sorry to say – an extraordinary *relief*. How wonderful to be acting like a real human being.

Who was it they were calling a saint?

The relief, however, is short-lived. Reality soon hits when you realize that the co-carer(s) onto whom you offloaded your angst are now even less likely to help.

The family mediator they don't have on *their* shoulder would, of course, whisper to them, 'Could she have had reason to explode/go chilly/drip sarcasm? Shouldn't you ring back and apologize, or at least suggest a way around the problem?'

Instead, into their ear, their furious child is whispering 'If that's the thanks you get when you offer to help, sod her, let her beg.' Or 'I was willing to help but she just wants it all her own way. There's no reasoning with her.'

This, of course, is quite a relief to them. If it is *your* fault, after all, then they are off the hook. (I once sat on a train next to a man who told me – straight-faced – that he no longer offers his sister help with their demented father because she 'always explodes at me for *no reason*.')

It is easy to see how a few years of this can produce such a store of resentment on both sides that resuming normal family relationships can seem impossible.

I have no solution. But I can, perhaps, offer both carers and carers' family members a list of things to do and not to do: you might, having read my list, think of suggestions yourself. If so, please go to the Keeping Mum site and add your own. Other carers will welcome any non-incendiary suggestions you might have to make.

Carers	
What to Do	**What Not to Do**
Ask for help in advance so family members can organize their diaries.	*Think you can do it alone;* you know it's not possible.
Allow family members their say: you don't have the monopoly on your piglet.	*Spurn offers of help because they don't fit your agenda.* Isn't there *anything* you can do with them?
Listen to suggestions. You never know, they might help.	*Fail to apologize* if you have let your furious child set the agenda.
Identify your non-negotiables and ask for help in achieving them.	*Assume family members are too busy/ unwilling to help:* people sometimes don't realize help is needed.
Remember, you are worth it. If you suffer from low self-esteem, do something about it. Why add to your problems? Ask your local Carers' Centre if they do assertiveness classes. If not, check at the local library or ask your GP.	*Keep quiet about your woes.* If things are getting difficult, *tell someone.* Actually, tell *everyone.* You cannot do it alone.
Plan for fun. If no one can cover this week's visit to the cinema with friends, say 'yes' instead for next week (and the week after).	*Keep battling on* – especially when you know you need a break.
Be sensitive to the fact that when family members are covering for you, their own projects are on hold.	*Isolate yourself.* If your family don't ring you, ring them.
Delegate things you don't have time for (like making sure you're getting the benefits to which you are entitled).	*Use being the main carer as a moral trump card.* Imagine how irritating this must be.

Carers' Family Members	
What to Do	**What Not to Do**
Make suggestions sensitively 'I was wondering if … would help? What do you think?', 'I have a friend who used to … do you think it would work with Dad?', 'I was going to try this, but wanted to check with you.'	*Criticize.* You might be absolutely right that the carer should have done this or that. But they won't thank you for telling them.
Ask how you might help and try to fit the carer's agenda; it's not, after all, *their* agenda.	*Assume they haven't thought of something*, especially if it is fairly obvious. If they are not doing it, there'll be a reason.
Commit to specific times/dates. Otherwise your offers of help are useless.	*Get irritated if asked to help unexpectedly.* The carer dislikes emergencies as much as you do.
Be sensitive to the carer's situation. It's not just your joint piglet you are supporting here.	*Leave the carer to get on with it.* A regular telephone call lets the carer know they are not completely alone.
Read a couple of books on caring/by carers and try to imagine how you would feel if you were the main carer.	*Fail to apologize* if you have let your furious child set the agenda.
Be understanding especially in the presence of the carer's furious child, however it manifests itself.	*Treat the carer as your equal.* The carer is operating with a serious handicap. They often can't do things you think they should do.
Go the extra mile. After all, this is what they are doing for your joint piglet.	*Offload your problems onto the carer* unless you are sure the carer is up to it.
Listen – particularly to silences; the tether's end is never far away.	*Assume the carer is managing.* Even if they seem to be, it's worth asking.
	Use blackmail by getting at the carer through your joint piglet.
	Forget that if the carer wasn't doing what they do, your joint piglet would have to go into a home, and/or someone else would have to do or pay for their care … you?

The Practicalities: Money, Property and the Law

First things first: I am neither a financial advisor nor a lawyer. If anything here strikes you as useful, get it checked by a professional. Nothing I say should be taken as the definitive guide to anything: your piglet(s), and the situation in which you are caring for them, may differ completely from my situation with my piglet. Remember, too, that the law and public policy are in constant flux – all the more reason to check things out thoroughly.

Having issued all these warnings, I hope you'll find some of this useful: it represents knowledge and understanding that I, and my carer friends, wish we'd had.

In this section we'll be looking at:

- **Lasting Powers of Attorney:** why you and your piglet need LPAs

- **The Court of Protection:** what happens to the carers of piglets without LPAs

- **Continuing care:** the importance of being assessed

- **Property ownership:** why joint house-ownership can be piglet-unfriendly

- **Varying wills:** how to change someone's will after they are dead

- **Appointeeships:** how to manage your piglet's pension and benefits

- **Selling property:** selling your piglet's house

- **Bank accounts:** day-to-day management of your piglet's money

- **Credit cards:** using your piglet's credit cards

- **Cash:** your piglet's handling of it

- **Direct Payments:** why your joy should be tempered with caution.

If you think anything I say is now outdated or plain wrong, or if you have better or different suggestions, it would be great if you'd get in touch (see the Resources chapter). Thank you in advance.

Lasting Powers of Attorney

If your piglet has no Lasting Power of Attorney (or Enduring Power of Attorney, as it was known before 1st October 2007) and is not yet completely mentally incapacitated, get them to a solicitor as quickly as possible. You really need a valid LPA.

LPAs come in two forms. One covers property and financial affairs, and replaces the Enduring Power of Attorney. The other covers health and welfare, and replaces the Living Will (we'll talk more about this kind in the next chapter). Both documents identify a trusted person as an 'attorney', giving them the power to make decisions on behalf of the 'donor' (the person whose LPA it is).

Many people fear that in completing an LPA they are losing control. If this is your piglet, it might be worth telling them that:

1. an LPA becomes active only when registered with the Office of the Public Guardian;

2. they can identify a 'named person' who must be notified of the registration and can object if they believe the donor is still mentally competent;

3. a certificate (within the form) must be signed by someone at the making of the LPA to attest to their belief that the donor is not under pressure.

Your piglet might also be susceptible to the fact that your life as a carer without an LPA will be intolerable. You will be at the mercy of the Court of Protection. This will cost your piglet much more than it costs to make and register an LPA. It will cost you, as their carer, your sanity.

The fact that you are a carer does not, of course, protect you from strokes, heart attacks, stray buses or lightning strikes. Fine (perhaps) if these things kill you and you have a will. But what if *you* become mentally incompetent? You need an LPA too.

The Court of Protection

When Dad had his stroke he had a will but no Enduring Power of Attorney. His will, as he wasn't dead, was useless. He had to be made a ward of the Court of Protection. I was appointed his 'Receiver', and as such became responsible for all his finances. These days you would be called a 'Deputy'. Under the supervision of the Court, you will receive and disburse your piglet's income, manage their investments and savings, and complete their tax returns and all their other financial documentation. You will have to account to the Court for everything you do.

The Court will make an Order setting out the powers and duties you have. You are required to carry out those duties 'sensitively, rigorously and responsibly' whilst:

- making only those decisions authorized by the Court;

- adhering to the five statutory principles of the Mental Capacity Act 2005;

- acting always in the person's best interests;

- applying 'certain standards of care and skill' in your decision-making; and

- having regard to all relevant guidance in the Code of Practice.

If you fail in any of these duties, you are liable to prosecution. You are required to pay a bond (likely to be in the region of £200) in case you fail in any of these duties. See the Resources chapter for some websites setting out the requirements and costs of the Court of Protection.

Here is my advice for dealing with the Court of Protection:

- Keep records of *everything*. Keep copies of all letters as well as dated contemporaneous notes of all telephone calls.

- Keep scrupulous records of every penny of your piglet's money that you spend.

- Familiarize yourself with the many charges the Court will apply. The website on page 279 will help.

- Check every bit of documentation that comes your way. File *all* of it.

- If you are unsure about anything, check. If necessary get independent legal or financial advice. Keep records of all such advice.

- Never make, and certainly don't implement, any decision unless and until you are certain you have the power to make it.

- Check every Court Order, especially the first one making you a Deputy, for errors. If (*IF?! Ha!*) you find one, ask immediately for a correction.

- Be patient: everything takes forever in Court of Protection land.

- Become word-perfect on the five principles of the Mental Capacity Act 2005, the Code of Practice, the 'duties and responsibilities' set out in the declaration you made as you became a Deputy, and the restrictions that apply to your particular Deputyship.

- You will be in breach of your Order if you fail to ensure your piglet gets all the benefits to which they are entitled.

- Always inform the Court of any relevant change in the situation of your piglet.

- Never rely on the assumption that the person you are talking to is sensible, intelligent, educated or well-meaning.

When you are at your lowest in your dealings with the Court, remember that you and the Court have something important in common: protecting your piglet's best interests. *YOU* know that your piglet doesn't need protecting from you. But they don't. It's their job to check up on you.

You will need a number of certified copies of the Order from the Court of Protection (or your piglet's property and financial affairs LPA). Every organization with which your piglet has financial dealings will need evidence that you are their Deputy/ attorney.

Continuing Care

You would think, wouldn't you, that if your piglet needs to go into a home because they have dementia, that they are going into the home because they are ill. Well, wouldn't you? But not every Council sees it like this every time. In fact, it's difficult not to think that Councils everywhere – especially in these cash-strapped times – are actively trying to convince carers that piglets with dementia are not *ill*, they just need social care.

The difference is important. To the extent that a piglet is *ill*, the care they need will be provided by the NHS. Free. To the extent that a piglet is *not* ill, but just elderly and frail, the care they need must be provided by the Council – and guess who gets to pay for most of it? That's right. Your piglet does.

If you do not realize the importance of this difference, you may find yourself paying for care that the NHS ought to pay for (and that your piglet *has* paid for in paying their National Insurance).

What you need to insist on is a 'continuing care assessment'. This should be – but often isn't – provided automatically, especially if your piglet is being discharged from hospital. The assessment will use a checklist to assess your piglet's competencies in a number of 'care domains'.

For further information there's a very helpful site from the Alzheimer's Society: see the Resources chapter.

Property Ownership

Mum and Dad, like many couples, owned their house jointly and had 'mirror wills', each leaving their share of the house and other property to the other.

The arrangement had obvious benefits. But as soon as Dad had his major stroke, the benefits became less obvious. Dad's stroke made it likely that he would, at some point, go into a nursing home.

When someone goes into a nursing home their income, assets and state of health (see 'Continuing Care', above) are assessed to determine their contribution to the fees of that nursing home. The value of any house they own (or part-own) will be taken into account except in certain very specific conditions.

One of those conditions is met if a spouse lives in the house. So long as Mum still lived in the house she and Dad owned, the value of the house was discounted for the purposes of calculating Dad's contribution to nursing home fees. There was never any possibility, whilst Mum was alive and living in the house, that Mum would have to sell the house to pay Dad's fees.

If Mum had died, though, while Dad was in the nursing home, their mirror wills and joint ownership would have made Dad sole owner of the house. The whole value of the house would then have been taken into account in calculating Dad's contribution. It is probable that all the proceeds from the sale of the house would have ended up in the hands of the nursing home.

To avoid this, our solicitor severed the joint tenancy of the house, making my parents 'tenants in common'. This meant that instead of Mum and Dad owning the whole house jointly, they each owned half of the house. Ownership of half a house makes possible bequeathing that half of the house to someone other than the person who owns the other half of the house.

At the same time, Mum's 'mirror will' was destroyed and a new one made (at that point Mum was still mentally competent) leaving Mum's share of the house to her children. Had Mum died while Dad was in the nursing home, Dad would not therefore have become sole owner of the house. He would have continued to own only half of it. We would have owned the other half. Only Dad's half of the house would have been counted in the calculation of his contribution to nursing-home fees.

There is nothing illegal in this. It is sensible financial planning. Dad would have paid his full whack of nursing-home fees, but his children would have inherited Mum's share of their house.

By law (and quite reasonably) a partner must be notified of the severing of a joint tenancy. This meant that Dad had to be given a letter informing him of it. His bewilderment – and inchoate grasp of the obvious importance of this step – was deeply painful for him and for me.

Be warned that any move of this kind might have implications for inheritance tax.

Varying Wills

A 'last Will and Testament' needn't be the final word on the distribution of property after death. A Will can be 'varied' – i.e. altered – any time in the two years following death, so long as all the beneficiaries to the Will agree.

When Dad died, his Will was finally activated. Mum, therefore, became the sole owner of their house. By then Mum had been diagnosed with Alzheimer's. I was determined she wouldn't go into a home. But I didn't see why, if she did, Dad's half of the house should be forfeited for nursing-home fees when this could – legally – be avoided.

My siblings and Mum agreed. As the five of us were the only beneficiaries under Dad's Will, this meant our solicitor could draw up a 'deed of variation' ensuring that Dad's half of the house was left to us, the children, rather than to Mum.

For the rest of the time Mum lived in the house, therefore, it was half-owned by her children. If she had gone into a nursing home at that point, only *her* half of the house would have gone to paying fees. Once again Mum would have paid her whole whack of nursing-home fees. But her children would have inherited Dad's share of their house.

There are again implications for inheritance tax. But here another warning is relevant: people who live in houses part-owned by their children are reliant on the goodwill of those children, and the spouses of those children. Do not underestimate the lure of money: even if the children are well behaved, what about their spouses? Are any divorces looming? To learn more, put 'deed of variation' into a search engine such as Google.

Appointeeships

If your piglet's only source of income is the State pension and various State benefits, you can apply to the Department of Work and Pensions (DWP) for an appointeeship. You might want to do this even if you have an LPA. It is very easy to set up and gives you the right to receive their pension and other benefits and to use the money for their benefit. You will also have to complete and sign forms on their behalf and make sure they get all the benefits to which they are entitled.

Much of the advice outlined above for interacting with the Court of Protection applies here. In particular, keep careful records and inform the DWP of any change in your piglet's circumstances.

You should also check *everything*. I once failed to notice that they had recorded as *annual* a small *quarterly* pension of Mum's. By the time this was noticed we had been overpaid £1,500. It took a great deal of hard work (and anxiety) on my part to persuade the pension people that, because I had been scrupulous in notifying them of changes, it wasn't our fault and they couldn't claw it back.

Trying to keep track of the benefits to which your piglet is entitled is an unending job. I found that keeping the pensions and benefits people informed of even the smallest change in Mum's situation was the only realistic way of doing this. It's labour-intensive, but at least you don't inadvertently break the law.

Selling Property

Trying to sell another person's house is no fun. If that person has dementia, it is even less fun. If they live 200 miles away, it is even worse. Without an LPA or an Order from the Court of Protection, your piglet will have to sign everything themselves. This will make your life hell.

Find all the documents you need before you start. If possible use a solicitor you know, trust and like. Brief the solicitor fully on the situation, and especially on the fact that your sale of the house is above board and legal despite the fact that your piglet – whose house it probably is – will deny all knowledge of it.

Ideally you should also know, trust and like your estate agent. Choose one, if you can, who can handle your bursting into tears on their shoulder. Make sure they understand that your piglet will express astonishment and concern every time the house-sale is mentioned. Make sure the estate agent can and will soothe your piglet's fear that they are being made homeless.

Arrange for your piglet to be out when people are shown round. People tend not to buy houses they think are being sold against the wishes of a poor confused old lady.

Brief the neighbours, the milkman, the postman, the cleaner and everyone else your piglet is likely to interact with. Then they won't, with excellent intentions, put serious spanners in the works. It is A GOOD THING that the police come to help little old ladies whose houses are being sold by wicked strangers. But you really do not need this.

If there's any chance you can send your piglet away for a week or a fortnight and clear the house in one go, then do it. I went down every weekend for months to sort through 61 years' worth of stuff. I did it while Mum was there. This made her desperately insecure and necessitated my explaining everything hundreds of times over. It also led to arguments. *Everything*, down to the tenth identical empty coffee jar, was, Mum insisted, central to her future happiness and security.

I don't know how I stayed sane.

Bank Accounts

During the years I cared for Mum, both from a distance and when she lived with me, I often had reason – believe it or not – to be hugely grateful to my bank. Isn't that amazing? So now, with gratitude, great pleasure … and the assurance they are not paying me (though if you happen to be the Chairman, CEO or any other bigwig from my bank and would like to thank me for this free publicity, please don't hesitate to get in touch. Cheques accepted.) … I name them: *FIRST DIRECT*.

They were truly fantastic. Every time I rang them, whether in the middle of the night or at Sunday lunchtime (carers must do it when they can), not only did a person answer the phone (usually immediately), that person was unfailingly polite, helpful and often asked me how my day was going. If I had a question, they would either answer it immediately or they would promise to ring back with the answer asap. Do you know what? They did. Every time.

Regularly, during the years I cared for Mum, I thanked my lucky stars that I had been able, before she became officially mentally incapacitated, to get her to transfer her accounts to First Direct, and to set up a Third Party Mandate in my name.

I cannot overemphasize the usefulness of this.

Thanks to this mandate, and the efficiency of First Direct, I was able to operate Mum's accounts by telephone as easily as I was able to operate my own. I arranged to have her pensions and benefits paid into her account, and from it I paid all her bills (by direct debit) and drew out cash to use on her behalf.

When Mum was finally awarded Direct Payments I was able, in the twinkling of an eye, to set up a new and separate account for them to be paid into. The Council's direct payment advisor, who was sitting with me, couldn't believe how easy it was.

The running of Mum's accounts was the only thing in the ten years that I cared for Mum that ran without a hitch and even with a certain amount of pleasure. If only I could have done the same with Dad.

Credit Cards

Ahem ... I am slightly worried about this. I am not sure it is legal. Having set up Mum's PIN myself, I simply used Mum's credit cards as if I were Mum.

You can see, can't you, why the Court of Protection is needed to protect piglets against unscrupulous carers? You can also see why an LPA, conferring authority on a person you trust, is such a useful safeguard. It was only because I had Mum's EPA (the forerunner of the LPA) that I was able to set up her PIN.

Cash

If your piglet is living with you, this is not much of a problem. They don't need much cash. But if you are caring from a distance, this can get difficult. Mum started to hide money. Then she wouldn't remember where she had hidden it. She always claimed not to have any. I had to conduct a thorough search of all her hiding places every time I went to stay.

I found the only sensible thing to do was set up accounts in all the shops Mum used, pay them myself, and then pay myself back from Mum's money.

Another reason you might hesitate to let your piglet have large amounts of money or a cheque book is that they might – as Mum did – spend it responding to all the 'special offers' that came to her by post (see page 9). I dealt with this by getting her mail redirected to me and sending the scam letters – literally hundreds of them – to the Trading Standards people.

Keep a careful eye on your piglet's bills and bank accounts. On at least two occasions Mum signed documents changing her energy suppliers, messing up all her direct debit arrangements.

Make sure all your family know that you are dealing with your piglet's financial arrangements. My niece – with excellent intentions – helped Mum get her pension paid into the post office account just after I had just succeeded in getting it paid into her bank account. It took a nifty bit of footwork to sort that one out.

Direct Payments, Individual and Personal Budgets

When things are getting serious, you or your piglet may qualify for Direct Payments. These are payments made by the Council to enable you to buy in the help you or your piglet has been assessed as needing. If you have read the blogs you will see that I was awarded £403 per week.

There are numerous restrictions on the way you can use the money, and you have to account for every penny of it. You can choose to have your Direct Payments managed by someone appointed by the Council, or you can choose to do it yourself.

Be warned: if your situation is serious enough to qualify you for Direct Payments, then you should think very seriously indeed about deciding to manage them yourself. In my case it proved the final straw. You really don't need to add advertising for, interviewing and/or setting up contracts to your workload. Be warned: the Government aims to get everyone eligible into 'personalized care' (which involves either Direct Payments or individual or personal budgets, which are subtly different) very soon because they cut down on the administration the Council must do. Well, of course they do. *You* do the admin instead.

On the other hand, these do allow you to decide what care you need and when: how you judge the autonomy versus extra work issue is, of course, up to you.

By the time you qualify for Direct Payments you will have a dedicated care manager. He or she will – I hope – guide you through the maze. You might also like to use the various carers' discussion boards (see the Resources chapter) to ask for advice.

This is an important step. Don't – as I did – let the relief of being given money to buy in care make you think your problems are over. Get as much advice as you can. You might start by checking out this page at the Carers UK website: http://www.carersuk.org/Information/Directpayments/Frequentlyaskedquestions

Looking Forward

I hope you have found some of these suggestions useful. I'm sure you will, now or later, have your own tips. You would be doing everyone a real favour if you would go to the Keeping Mum website (see the Resources chapter) and put them in the relevant section.

In the next chapter we'll take a look at the practicalities around your piglet's health and welfare issues.

More Practicalities: Social Services, Health and Welfare

I am not a doctor, care worker or social worker. As a carer, though, I have had 14 years' worth of experience of dealing with those who are. I also have lots of friends who have between them a huge amount of experience. This section is based on the things we wish we had known. I hope you find it helpful. But don't take anything I say below as more than a guide. Always consult the professionals.

In this section we'll be looking at:

- **Health and welfare Lasting Powers of Attorney:** why health and welfare LPAs might be useful

- **Medical matters:** managing your piglet's health

- **Social services:** getting help for yourself and your piglet

- **Day care:** getting your piglet settled in day care

- **Respite care:** securing and managing respite care for yourself and your piglet

- **A good death:** your piglet's last wishes.

As with the previous chapter, if you think that anything I say is unhelpful or plain wrong, or if you have better or different suggestions, it would be kind of you to let me know. Thank you in advance!

Lasting Powers of Attorney

Under the Mental Capacity Act 2005, every adult is presumed to have the capacity to make their own decisions – however unwise – unless it is proven they cannot do so.

This means that anyone caring for the health and welfare of your piglet has a duty to respect their autonomy. They are also required to respect your piglet's confidence.

This will make life impossible for you as a carer unless you have a health and welfare LPA giving your piglet's permission for you to be told what you need to know, and for others to be able to act on the decisions you make.

In completing this LPA your piglet has a lot of discretion in deciding how much power to give you. They must make a conscious decision, for example, about whether to give you the right to refuse, on their behalf, treatment that would keep them alive.

The safeguards mentioned on page 237 apply also in the case of these LPAs.

Medical Matters

In caring for your piglet you will find yourself dealing with memory clinic doctors, your piglet's GP, the community psychiatric nurse, their dentist, optician and chiropodist, the hearing-aid people, the mobility people, occupational therapists and many others.

It is to the credit of such people that they often insist on speaking directly to your piglet. Unfortunately, you and I know that your piglet will lie through their teeth, telling the doctor they take no medication, the optician they can see perfectly, and the dentist they brush their teeth thrice daily. You can't, of course, contradict your piglet because you respect their dignity too much.

I used to write out the information I believed to be relevant and give the written note to the receptionist to pass on to the doctor. This saves your having to gesticulate behind your piglet's back. Sometimes I told Mum I had an appointment after her, and asked the receptionist to keep an eye on Mum during my private consultation. Be careful, though: I once lost Mum in a busy hospital.

One day your piglet will no longer be able to respond to instructions or answer questions. This makes it difficult to discover what's wrong with them. One day some nice medics will devise diagnostic tests that can be applied to people with dementia. Until then it is often hit and miss.

You can help by having as complete a medical history for your piglet as you can. You need to start on this before your piglet's memory goes completely. Old diaries might help.

The healthier the regime you keep your piglet on, the less likely it is that they'll ever need serious medical intervention. Given the difficulties attending such interventions you may one day be glad you kept them fit and well even as their mind fragmented. A good night's sleep, regular exercise, nutritious food, regular hydration and scrupulous personal hygiene all help.

Piglets do not like dental examinations. Supervise regular tooth-brushing. Cut down your piglet's sugar intake. Would sugar-free chewing gum work for your piglet?

Don't forget the annual flu jab. Do you really need your piglet feeling dreadful for ten days? Get yours, too: what would happen if you were out for the count for ten days?

I gave my doctor a supply of stamps so I could renew prescriptions by phone and have them sent to the local chemist, who delivered. Buy yourself a pill dispenser. It avoids confusion about which pills your piglet has had and when.

Keep a health logbook: bowel motions, medication, walks, meals, instances of sickness ... all useful information if the doctor has to be called. Send it with your piglet to day care so it is a complete record.

Make sure your details are on all your piglet's records. Preferably in red. You also want the fact you are a carer recorded on *your* medical records. Your doctor should have a list of people to contact in case of emergency. I wouldn't have known what to do if my doctor had not, one day, used this list to get my sister to take over.

Social Services

You are legally entitled to a carer's assessment as soon as you care, or will soon have to care, for someone for a 'substantial amount of time' on a 'regular basis'. I let someone on my Council dissuade me and so missed out on many benefits.

The assessment will enable you to discuss with a professional the support – practical, physical, emotional and psychological – you need to enable you to care. You will be able to reflect on how you will continue to work, care for your family and have a social life.

In principle you may be able to get help with practical tasks (meals, personal care, telecare services such as alarm buttons and movement sensors), aids and equipment (e.g. mobility and bath aids), and possibly even home alterations (convert a downstairs room to a bedroom, add a bathroom), advice on benefits, day care and respite care and money in the form of Direct Payments, Independent Living Allowance personal budgets or care vouchers. Check out the websites of the carers' organizations (see Resources pages 275–84) and seek advice on the chat zones.

Dedicated care managers are worth their weight in gold. They keep a personal eye on you, regularly assess your situation, ensure you and your piglet get the benefits to which you are entitled and help you through the different stages. Eventually they will negotiate your piglet's move into a nursing home.

Day Care

If your piglet is sociable, they will enjoy day care. You will certainly enjoy day care. Day care centres are usually open from 10 until 3. This doesn't allow for proper days out, but it gives you a breather. You can go out for lunch, read a book or watch a bit of daytime television. You might even do a few chores, or get a part-time job. Anything that'll keep you sane.

I went with Mum to her first day at day care. It gave me the confidence to leave her there. Mum started by going twice a week and graduated to four times a week. For me it was a life-saver. At first it gave me a break. Then, as Mum deteriorated, I was able to check my intuitions against those of the care workers, and secure advice from people who knew Mum almost as well as I did.

The day care centre people need to know about special diets and their implications. It is also useful for them to know of any significant likes or dislikes. You might write a short biography of your piglet, laminate it and give it to the manager of your piglet's day care centre.

If your piglet's day care centre is Council-run, your piglet will probably be entitled to transport. If so, they'll be collected by a special bus and returned at the end of the day. A care worker always accompanies them. This is extremely useful. But if I had been able to drive at the time I would have preferred to take Mum to day care and collect her myself rather than have her sit in a bus being driven around collecting other people for up to two hours, twice a day. I am sure this added to her confusion.

You might like to check out whether weekend day care is available in your area. This can facilitate something approaching a normal social and family life for you. I was delighted, when Mum started Saturday day care, to be able to go to weddings again (so long as they were local). What's really needed, of course, is evening care.

Oh, well, we can dream …

Respite Care

Do not accept the first place offered for respite care. If you can, check out a few and choose the best. The same thing applies to adult placements (where a family or a single person will have you piglet to stay for the odd weekend, a day here or there, or even a full week).

Check, in particular, on the arrangements for respite residents. Some homes have dedicated beds. Others put respite piglets into whichever rooms they have available. Whichever is the case, respite residents need to be carefully monitored, especially at night. You don't want your sleepless piglet to wander unchecked in a strange place.

If your piglet is going for adult placement, make sure they have stair gates, bath grips, night lights and other safety features, and that your piglet's bedroom is near that of their host(ess), and the lavatory.

Are respite residents expected to use a commode? If so, consider buying a commode and using it at home for a few weeks so your piglet gets used to it. If there is an en-suite in the respite room can the light be left on overnight?

You might like to check out the reports on the possible homes written by the Care Quality Commission, whose job it is to see that national standards are met (see the Resources chapter). See if the home will allow your piglet to go to them for day care for the weeks leading up to their respite week. Go with them and do what you can to make them familiar with the place.

It might be worth treating your first couple of weeks' respite as trial runs. Accept that you will get no respite during them, but that you'll dedicate these trial runs to making sure you get decent respite in future. Spend some part of each day with your piglet, and be there to tuck them in at night. It'll be worth it if your piglet settles in happily.

Find out from the home what your piglet needs to bring with them. I assumed – wrongly – that the home would supply shampoo and soap. Do not send anything precious. Keep an inventory of everything you send. The home will make their own inventory. Make sure it tallies with yours. Name *everything* with indelible ink.

I hope respite works for you.

Nursing Homes

When your piglet has lost their language, their ability to feed and entertain themselves and their continence, it is almost certainly better that they be cared for by professionals. Your care manager will help you complete the forms needed for a proper assessment. The assessment you need here is the one for continuing care (see page 240). If your piglet's dementia is serious, their fees might be paid for by the NHS. Don't forget to seek advice from carers' organizations or from carers' chat zones.

Do not think that your piglet's going into a home means that you are no longer involved in their care. Most nursing homes are only too happy for you to come in and help with your piglet. Some carers almost move into the home, at least until they are happy their piglet is being cared for.

Preparation

The notes above on preparing for respite care are also relevant in preparing your piglet to go into a nursing home. Quite often, though, the move into a nursing home is an emergency measure when something happens to upset existing arrangements. In many cases, as in mine, a move to a nursing home is mandated by the carer's suddenly finding themselves unable to cope.

The way of avoiding this, of course, is not to allow yourself to get to this stage.

I understand that the SPECAL system (see Oliver James' book *Contented Dementia**) insists that those who sign up accept explicitly, at the time of signing, that their piglet will eventually go into a home. I think this is a good idea. It helps carers avoid the feeling that their piglet's going into a home is a failure on their part.

Choosing a Care Home

You may not have a great deal of choice about the home your piglet goes into. If you are able to choose, then do not do so until after you have watched the programme 'Can Gerry Robinson Fix Dementia Care Homes?' There's a link in the Resources chapter about where you can get this. It will give you a much better idea of what a good home looks like (and sadly, what a bad one looks like).

At the very least you should check out the Care Quality Commission's report on the care homes you are looking at. (You'll find the CQC's contact details in the Resources chapter).

You will probably be surprised, once your piglet goes into a nursing home, just how quickly they become institutionalized. This is a good thing. Your role will then be that of visitor and occasional helper.

---

*James, Oliver, *Contented Dementia: 24-hour Wraparound Care for Lifelong Well-being* (Vermillion, 2009)

Visiting Your Piglet

Visiting someone in a nursing home can be tear-jerking, frustrating or worrying. Mostly it is boring. Your piglet probably can't hold a decent conversation, and neither can the other inmates. The nurses and care workers are busy.

Think about giving your piglet a manicure or pedicure, a head massage or a hand or shoulder rub. Maybe you could wash their hair for them? Take them for a walk around the grounds. Look at picture books. Perhaps they would even like to go for a drive? I used to visit at mealtimes so I could be sure that Mum was eating enough. Some piglets are able to come home for tea occasionally. My friend Philippa once brought her husband Martin home for Christmas (she paid for a nurse to come, too).

You might consider joining the families committee and having a say in how the home is run. If you are not a committee person, keep an eye on noticeboards. Here you should see notification of visits from hairdressers, chiropodists and other professionals who might be useful to your piglet. You'll probably have to add your piglet's name to a list. If you don't see a service offered that you know your piglet would like, make enquiries.

Never be afraid to make suggestions to the home about how they might improve the care they provide. For example, does your piglet's home allow – or, better, *expect* – piglets to help? Piglets can fold laundry, lay tables, help make beds … If not, why not suggest it?

Most homes have facilities for residents to attend religious services. They also have activities like poster-painting, music therapy and keep fit. Mum *adored* music therapy, which consisted largely in making rhythmic noises to piano accompaniment. A good sing-song always went down well in Mum's home. If residents spend all day sitting around, then suggest a few activities.

Check out the medical care your piglet will have available in the home. Will the home use your piglet's own GP, or will they have to register with a new one? The home will usually deal with all prescriptions and medications, but check they have the right drugs on their lists. Make sure the home is aware of any allergies.

Make a collage of photographs for your piglet's door, or write a short biography to laminate and pin on it. Make sure it gives a flavour of what your piglet was like in their prime. Include any major successes your piglet has had in life. Talk to the care workers about your piglet and what they were like.

Personalize your piglet's room. But remember to name everything, especially those things you'd one day like back.

A Good Death

Once your piglet is in a home you will want to make sure the home can always contact you. It might be worth having a dedicated pay-as-you-go mobile to which only the home has the number. That way even if you turn off other phones for a bit of peace, that one can be left on. I didn't do this and have often cringed since at the thought I might have had the phone turned off when the final call came. I feel privileged to have been with Mum for her last night. If the home hadn't been able to get hold of me …

Check out also the arrangements the home has for dealing with life-threatening incidents. Do they keep morphine or other effective pain relief on the premises? If not, how is effective pain relief administered in the case of an emergency? If you read the blog you might remember that Mum's home did not have adequate pain relief for her on her last night. It had never occurred to me to ask.

Rehearse in your mind the phone call that will tell you that a life-threatening incident has happened. This will not prevent you from being hugely shocked, but it might help you do sensible things. Perhaps you could keep a small bag packed so you can grab it in case of emergencies? On Mum's last night I wished I had had the foresight to do that.

I was so glad, on Mum's final night, to have lodged with her nursing home a copy of her 'Living Will'. (Mum's mental incapacity pre-dated the LPA era.) This directed those treating her not to prolong her life if, at the time of a life-threatening incident, she was suffering from dementia and/or an incurable illness that was causing (or would cause) unrelievable pain or otherwise significantly reduce the quality of her life. It also appointed me as someone who would make the final decision on her behalf.

Had the nursing home not had this document (or had I chosen not to act on it) they would have had to rush Mum by ambulance into hospital on her final night. There she might have been subjected to the indignity of vigorous life-prolonging treatment whilst I looked on helplessly.

They might even have succeeded in prolonging her life. I adored my lovely Mum. But I saw no point, on the night she died, in prolonging her life. It would have been cruel.

A health and welfare LPA is one way for your piglet to indicate their wishes on life-sustaining treatment, and their choice of a person to make decisions on their behalf. But it is still possible, I understand, to use the less formal document Mum had. It is called an 'advance directive' or 'Living Will'. If you have specified in such a document that you do not want life-sustaining treatment, then any doctor who provides it is subject to civil liability or criminal prosecution.

Advance directives, unlike health and welfare LPAs, cost nothing to make and are easy to draw up. The document has to be signed by at least one witness and it must contain certain things (such as the direction that it stands 'even if life is at risk'.)

If you go this route, make absolutely sure that the document you draw up satisfies all the legal requirements. Put 'Living Will' or 'advance directive' into a search engine like Google, and make sure the website whose guidance you accept is a reputable one. (The Government itself has such a site; see the Resources chapter.)

The effect of your piglet's having refused life-sustaining treatment is that this treatment will not be given. If your piglet develops a lung infection they will not be given antibiotics. If they have a stroke they will not be given life support. If they have a heart attack they will not be given cardio-pulmonary resuscitation.

Make sure you are ready for this.

I hope you have found some of these suggestions useful. Remember that everyone has their own way of caring, and if any of these suggestions strike you as unnecessary/useless or whatever, then please do ignore them! If you have your own tips please visit the Keeping Mum website (see the Resources chapter) and add them to the relevant section.

Checklists for the Different Stages of Caring

Checklists

These checklists result from reflections on what I and my carer-friends *wish* we'd done. None of us did everything. You won't either (probably). But I hope they help.

In the Beginning (1)

If your piglet has been diagnosed with a dementia, like Alzheimer's, which develops relatively slowly, here are a few things to consider:

- Try to persuade your piglet to complete Lasting Powers of Attorney (see pages **236–37**).

- Help them to caption photographs of the family.

- Compile a complete medical history of your piglet and their family.

- Suggest your piglet writes their life story.

- Find a solicitor you like and trust.

- Find a fee-charging financial advisor you like and trust. (Commission-charging advisors have an incentive to sell you things you don't need.) See the Resources chapter.

- Start acquiring skills – car maintenance, family finance – for which you rely on your piglet.

- Read the money pages for articles on caring and/or mental incapacity.

- Research your piglet's dementia, its developmental stages and likely timeline.

- Brainstorm with family on realistic options for care under different contingencies.

- If moving house is likely, start disposing of things and find an estate agent you like.

- Start your piglet thinking about giving up driving.

- If you don't drive, start learning.

- If you intend to use SPECAL (see Oliver James *Contented Dementia*, Vermillion Press, 2009) start now.

It's likely you'll have a year or so to do these things, and so make the future easier.

In the Beginning (2)

If your piglet becomes demented overnight, you will be exhausted and in emotional turmoil. But if you can find some energy, you might:

- Register your piglet's Lasting Powers of Attorney (LPAs) with the Office of the Public Guardian (see the Resources chapter)

- If there are no LPAs you need to find out about the Court of Protection (see page 237).

- Was your piglet in charge of finances? Can you pay their bills? Talk to their bank manager.

- Before your piglet is discharged from hospital learn as much as possible about their prognosis, treatment and care.

- If your piglet is incontinent, learn how to deal with it. (Check out the carers' chat zones: see the Resources chapter.)

- Do not assume you have to do the caring: mightn't a home be better?

- If your piglet is going into a home, get a Continuing Care assessment (see page **240**).

- Consider the implications of caring for your piglet at home. Will you need to adapt the house? Get some training? Can you do this before their discharge?

- You do not have to accept the first discharge date suggested if you are not ready.

- Join Carers UK or the Princess Royal Trust for Carers (see the Resources chapter).

- Notify your employers of your new situation if you intend to continue working.

- Get a carer's assessment from local Social Services.

- Check out the benefits to which you or your piglet are entitled (see the Resources chapter).

- Try not to make unilateral decisions: your decision-making ability is impaired.

- Accept help from friends, neighbours and family members.

- Talk to your GP about benefits and support.

In the Middle

Once the dementia has started to bite you will need support:

- Identify your non-negotiables. Aim not to give up the things that matter most.

- Brainstorm ways of getting them (see Tips for Carers, page **219**).

- Even if you think your piglet will hate day care it's worth a try.

- Call a family powwow; ask for help even if only for ideas about how to get help.

- Your employer must at least consider your working flexible hours. Check up on the rights you have as a working carer.

- If you don't use the internet, learn how; you'll find it invaluable (see the Resources chapter to get help).

- Put 'carers (your area)' into a search engine such as Google to learn about local care options.

- Make sure you and your piglet get the benefits to which you are entitled (see the Resources chapter).

- A dedicated care manager is a very good thing. Contact your local Council.

- You want to know *the minute* you are eligible for respite care. Your care manager will help.

- If you have a Carers' Centre visit them.

- Check out courses for carers. First aid, entertaining people with dementia and lifting (so you don't hurt your back) are all useful.

- Join a carers' group, either face-to-face or online, to meet other carers, make friends and learn a lot.

- Join Carers UK or the Princess Royal Trust for Carers. Get their factsheets. See the Resources chapter.

- Check whether you are entitled to a Council grant for modifying your house.

- Put 'carers' holidays' into a search engine (or look in the Resources chapter) and investigate holidays for carers and their piglets. You might be entitled to a grant (from the Council or the Carers' Centre).

- Ask your Council whether you are eligible for free travel when you are with your piglet.

- Join the media panels of the main carers' and dementia organizations. Help to tell everyone about what it's like to be a carer.

The End Stages

Things are grim. Your piglet can't be left alone and can do very little for themselves. They may be doubly incontinent. If they are fit and well, they need constant entertainment. You are exhausted and possibly lonely. I hope you belong to a carers' organization?

- Get your care manager's direct number and don't let them go away without telling you who is replacing them.

- Ideally your piglet will be going to day care three or four days a week. It's only from 9–3 (usually), but how else are you going to stay sane?

- You should now be getting respite care. If not, agitate for it.

- Ask your care manager about adult placement. It will give you a regular break: worth it just for the anticipation.

- Investigate whether there is a piglet transport system in your area. It'll save you the nightmare of public transport.

- Your piglet should be on the highest attendance allowance and is exempt from paying Council Tax.

- If you have altered your house check whether you are eligible for help with Council Tax.

- Ask Social Services to do a risk assessment of your house. Check out grants for alterations suggested.

- Are you eligible for Direct Payments or an individual allowance?

- Join a carers' group, either face-to-face or online. Ask other carers what they are getting/doing and what is helping them.

- Get help with the admin associated with Direct Payments or individual budgets (ask your care manager).

- Think about nursing homes. It will almost certainly have to happen. Check out a few, identify the best and make enquiries.

- Consult your care manager about putting your piglet on to the waiting list for a home. You can always refuse a place if you get to the top of the list before you are ready.

- Find out about funding for care homes. It isn't as bad as it sounds because your piglet's pension and benefits will go towards the fees.

- Get an assessment for continuing care (see page 240).

- Investigate the position *you* will be in if your piglet goes into a nursing home. You don't want to be taken by surprise.

You probably feel you spend your life fire-fighting. A nursing home is probably inevitable: try to see it as a natural progression.

Respite Care (or Adult Placement)

Respite care was a disaster for me. I was desperately in need of it and didn't prepare properly. This checklist is based on what I wish I had done.

- Don't leave respite until you get desperate and are unable to prepare.

- Spend time in the respite place with your piglet. Will they take your piglet for day care before the respite week so they can get used to it?

- Are the bedrooms used for respite near a nursing station? How soon will a wandering piglet be intercepted? How often are respite residents monitored during the night?

- Try to get your piglet into the hearts of the care workers and nurses.

- Get a list of everything your piglet will need. Do they provide shampoo and soap, or must you?

- If your piglet will have to use a commode, might you get one to use at home to get your piglet used to it?

- See your first respite weeks as practice runs. Stay with your piglet during the day and tuck them in at night. If you can get respite to work you'll eventually be able to have completely free time.

- Make sure *someone* is on call during respite weeks. It needn't be you.

- Familiarize the home with your piglet's likes and dislikes, special diets etc.

- Do not pack anything you would be sorry to lose and keep a full inventory.

- Do not send originals of precious family photographs or anything you are not prepared to lose.

- Name *everything*: dentures, slippers, shampoo bottles, toothbrush, handkerchiefs …

- If you need to complain, get support. You won't have the energy to do it alone.

In a Home

OK, I know how you feel. Here's a BIG HUG (X). The respite care list will help with your piglet's needs. This is about what *you* need.

- Take time off. You need sleep. Be nice to yourself.

- Don't feel you need to visit all the time. Your piglet is in the hands of the professionals, they'll be looked after.

- Ensure the home has your piglet's Living Will, or health and welfare LPA.

- You were doing a HUGE job and suddenly you're not. Don't berate yourself for feeling at a loss.

- Go out for a coffee with others in the same position. Coffee? Hey – why not *dinner?* (It needn't be expensive – you can do it at home.) Talk about your piglets until you're in tears.

- If you can't get out, do it online.

- Tears are healing. Listen to sad music, think sad thoughts, have a wallow. It'll make you feel much better.

- When you visit your piglet, don't expect an ecstatic welcome (or even recognition). Read companionably to them (even if they are not listening).

- When you are up to it, brainstorm on what you're going to do with all your free time.

- Release some energy. Go for a long walk, hire a bike, punch a pillow.

- You probably don't do small talk yet. See only people who understand.

- You are still officially a carer and can continue to use Carers' Centres, go on outings and attend meetings. Let yourself down gently.

- Buy yourself a cheap mobile, give its number *only* to the nursing home and keep it with you at all times.

- Pack yourself a bag to grab in case you are called to the home and have to stay.

Soon your piglet will be institutionalized which, for them, is the best thing that can happen.

Death

The suggestions under 'In a Home' will be useful here too. A chapter in your life has closed and you need to mourn it as well as your piglet.

- If possible, sit with your piglet, talk to them, touch them, hold their hand.

- If you weren't able to be there, forgive yourself. Apparently people sometimes choose to die *because* their loved ones aren't there.

- You will probably feel relief as well as sorrow, guilt, puzzlement, anger, disbelief … just let it come.

- Get a copy of *What to Do When Someone Dies 2009: From Funeral Planning to Probate and Finance.* It'll tell you everything you need to know.

- The funeral arrangements will probably keep you busy. That's good.

- Don't do anything you don't want to do. People will (or should) understand. If you want to be alone, tell them. If you want a specific person, ring them.

- After the funeral you might feel worse. It is now that the real mourning starts.

- Remember that crying is good.

- Contact a bereavement support group. The Cruse helpline (0844 477 9400), will help you find a local group.

- Your fellow carers will help; don't hesitate to call on them.

- If you find yourself talking to your piglet, that's fine. I still talk to Mum occasionally.

Picking Up the Pieces

When the first wave of mourning is over you will – I hope – want to pick up the pieces of your life. If your piglet was in a home you may already have started this process. Don't be surprised if you have to start again.

- Don't expect to carry on immediately. Everything I did in the six months after Mum's death was useless. It would have been better to take time off.

- Solitary walking enabled me to think about Mum, myself and what I wanted to do.

- Resist the urge to volunteer your services elsewhere. You need a rest. I waited a year before volunteering for things.

- If you eventually volunteer to help other carers, expect to have to train. Being an expert on *your* piglet doesn't make you an expert on all piglets.

- With a friend brainstorm the things you'd like to do, and how to do them.

- Boost your self-esteem: acquire a new skill, take classes in something fascinating, volunteer for something enjoyable.

- Make new friends by attending evening classes, going to a new church or other place of worship, volunteering …

- Make yourself feel deliciously wicked. Mum took herself off for garlic mushrooms at the Little Chef. I get in a large pizza, pour a glass of red wine and watch a silly DVD.

- During carers' week hold a tea/dinner party and charge people to come, make and sell cakes, offer your services as a car mechanic …

I hope you find some of these suggestions useful. If you have others – and I am sure you do – please tell us about them on the Keeping Mum website (see the Resources chapter).

Afterword

I hope you have enjoyed reading this book. I hope, too, that you have found it helpful.

I am flourishing, now, as an independent person. I am getting to the point where I am ready to take on some voluntary work and I will almost certainly make use of my experience with dementia to do something for people with dementia and their carers.

Society is facing an explosion of mental health issues. There are currently about 750,000 people with dementia. This is expected to double over the next 30 years. For the first few years, at least, most of these people will be cared for by family members.

Carers are becoming more visible in society – but if you are a carer I'm sure you'll agree they are not yet visible enough. I shall do my best to make sure caring becomes more visible. But we have a long way to go. If you, like me, are an ex-carer, consider joining me in doing your best to make carers even more visible. If you are still a carer, register with a caring or dementia charity so they can use you as a case study … it's you and the care you give your piglet that'll get the message across more effectively than anything else.

Resources

Please visit the Keeping Mum website at www.keepingmum.
org.uk to get further exclusive content, sign up to hear more from
Marianne and become part of the Keeping Mum community.

General Information, Advice and Support for Carers

Carers Direct

www.nhs.uk/carersdirect/Pages/CarersDirectHome.aspx
0808 802 0202 (8 am to 9 pm Monday to Friday, 11 am to 4 pm
at weekends)
http://www.carersdirectenquiry.nhs.uk
Up-to-date information from the NHS.

Carers UK

20 Great Dover Street
London SE1 4LX
020 7378 4999
www.carersuk.org
Advice line: 0808 808 7777 (Wednesday and Thursday 10 am to
midday and 2 pm to 4 pm)
www.carersuk.org/Contactus

Directgov
www.direct.gov.uk/en/CaringForSomeone/index.htm
The Government's site for carers: very useful.

Helpguide.org
helpguide.org/elder/alzheimers_disease_dementia_support_
caregiver.htm
helpguide.org/contact.php
Excellent advice and support for carers of those with dementia.

The Princess Royal Trust for Carers
Unit 14, Bourne Court
Southend Road
Woodford Green
Essex
IG8 8HD
0844 800 4361
www.carers.org
Help Directory: www.carers.org/getting-help :
www.carers.org/contact-us

Advice and Information on Dementia

Alzheimer's Society
Devon House
58 St Katharine's Way
London E1W 1LB
020 7423 3500
www.alzheimers.org.uk
0845 300 0336 (8:30 am to 6:30 pm Monday to Friday)
enquiries@alzheimers.org.uk

Dementia UK
6 Camden High Street
London NW1 0JH
020 7874 7200
www.dementiauk.org
Admiral Nurses Direct: 0845 257 9406 (Tuesdays and Thursdays
11 am to 8:45 pm, Saturdays 10 am to 1 pm)
info@dementiauk.org

Information about Dementia on the Internet

From the NHS
www.nhs.uk/conditions/dementia/Pages/Introduction.aspx
www.nhs.uk/pathways/dementia/Pages/Landing.aspx

From the BBC
www.bbc.co.uk/health/physical_health/conditions/dementia1.
shtml

From BUPA
hcd2.bupa.co.uk/fact_sheets/html/dementia.html

Advice and Information for and on the Elderly

AgeUK
York House
207–221 Pentonville Road
London N1 9UZ
0800 107 8977
www.ageuk.org.uk
Advice line: 0800 169 6565
contact@ageuk.org.uk

Counsel and Care
Twyman House
16 Bonny Street
London NW1 9PG
0845 300 7585
www.counselandcare.org.uk
advice@counselandcare.org.uk
Advice and information for older people and their carers.

Independent Age
Independent Age
6 Avonmore Road
London W14 8RL
020 7605 4200
www.independentage.org.uk
charity@independentage.org.uk

Carers' Work and Finances

Carers and Work
www.carersuk.org/Information/Workandcaring

Citizens Advice Bureau
Myddelton House
115–123 Pentonville Road
London N1 9LZ
020 7833 2181
www.adviceguide.org.uk
Financial advice: www.citizensadvice.org.uk/index/partnerships/
generic_financial_advice.htm

Court of Protection

www.publicguardian.gov.uk/about/court-of-protection.htm – the website of the Court of Protection
www.lindermyers.co.uk/faqs-for-court-of-protection_757.html – an excellent website from a firm of solicitors offering information about the Court of Protection

National Centre for Independent Living

Unit 3.40
Canterbury Court
1–3 Brixton Road
London SW9 6DE
0207 587 1663
www.ncil.org.uk
Advice line: 0845 026 4748
nciluk.org/contact
Everything you need to know about Direct Payments and Individual Budgets

Office of the Public Guardian

0845 330 2900
www.publicguardian.gov.uk

Pensions Advisory Service

www.pensionsadvisoryservice.org.uk
0845 601 2923

Benefit Enquiry Line

0800 6060265

Online Financial Advice

Money Made Clear: www.moneymadeclear.org.uk/guides/
family/caring_for_someone.html
Paul Lewis (award-winning financial journalist): www.videojug.
com/interview/how-to-finance-care-for-elderly-parents
To help find an independent financial advisor: www.unbiased.
co.uk

Carers' Discussion Boards

www.carers.org/forums – the Princess Royal Trust for Carers
www.carersuk.org/Forums – Carers UK
www.chill4us.com/news/index.php – Chill4Us (by carers for
carers)
www.mencap.org.uk/discussion.asp?id=2275 – Mencap
www.alzheimers.org.uk/site/scripts/documents.
php?categoryID=200317 – Alzheimer's Society
www.youngcarers.net – for young carers, run by qualified youth
workers
www.ageuk.org.uk/chat2 – AgeUK

Holidays for Carers (with and without piglets)

www.tourismforall.org.uk/search.php?query=carers&search=1
www.carers.org/help-directory/taking-holiday
www.carersuk.org/Information/Helpwithcaring/Takingabreak

Information and Advice on Nursing Homes

Care Quality Commission
www.cqc.org.uk
03000 616161
www.cqc.org.uk/contactus/contactusonline.cfm
Information and advice about health and social care. This is
where to check out a possible nursing home. It is also where to
make a complaint.

Elderly Accommodation Council
EAC FirstStop Advice
3rd Floor
89 Albert Embankment
London SE1 7TP
0800 0099 66
www.housingcare.org
Advice Line: 0800 377 7070
info@firststopadvice.org.uk

'Can Gerry Robinson Fix Dementia Care Homes?' is available at
www.open2.net/healtheducation/health_socialcare/dementia/
index.html

For the 'This Is Me' leaflet: alzheimers.org.uk/site/scripts/
documents_info.php?documentID=1290

For Continuing Care information: alzheimers.org.uk/site/scripts/
documents_info.php?documentID=399

End of Life Care

For information about living wills: www.direct.gov.uk/en/
Governmentcitizensandrights/Death/Preparation/DG_10029429

End of Life Care
www.gsttcharity.org.uk/projects/eolc.html
www.nhs.uk/Planners/end-of-life-care/Pages/End-of-life-care.
aspx
www.endoflifecareforadults.nhs.uk

Bereavement Support

British Association for Counselling and Psychotherapy
0870 443 5219 (they will put you onto a local counsellor or
therapist)

Cruse
0844 477 9400

Samaritans
08457 909090

Guidance on arranging a funeral
www.gsttcharity.org.uk/whattodoafterdeath.html

Help with funeral costs
www.direct.gov.uk/en/Diol1/DoItOnline/DG_4017717

Pet Welfare and Bereavement

Care for pets after the death of owner:

RSPCA Home for Life
www.rspca.org.uk/getinvolved/supportus/leavealegacy/
homeforlife
0300 123 0239

Cinnamon Trust
www.cinnamon.org.uk
01736 7157900

Support after a pet dies:
Animal Samaritans
www.animalsamaritans.org.uk/bereave.htm
020 8303 1859

Blue Cross
www.bluecross.org.uk/2083/Pet-Bereavement-Support-Service.
html
0800 096 6606

Miscellaneous

Carers' World Radio
www.carersworldradio.com
0208 123 0652
A radio station dedicated to carers.

Dementia Services Development Centre
www.dementia.stir.ac.uk
Lots of practical information about living with dementia
including advice about organizing one's home.

Family Mediation
www.familymediationhelpline.co.uk
0845 602 627
info@familymediationhelpline.co.uk
Get help to stop that fury.

HDS
0800 043 0852
sales@hds-uk.com
Personal care products.

Volunteering England
www.volunteering.org.uk
Supports, enables and celebrates volunteering.

Whateverage
www.whateverage.co.uk
01588 680369
www.whateverage.co.uk/contact-us.aspx
Simple and reasonably priced guides to getting online, cheap
short courses for beginners and a helpline.